RISKY SEX

NATIONAL BEST SELLER

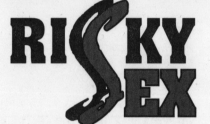

RISKY SEX

The Onslaught of Sexually Transmitted Diseases

Author - Stephen J Genuis M.D. F.R.C.S.(C), D.A.B.O.G.
Editor - Shelagh K Genuis B.Sc.O.T.
Illustration - Loren Chabot
Graphic Design and Production - Danie Hardie

KEG
Publishing

I dedicate this book to my dear wife, Shelagh. With her capable skills, she was often able to draw out and better articulate some of the ideas I have tried to present. We spent many hours pouring over certain areas and enjoying each other's company. The constant love and support she brings to our family provides the prerequisite environment necessary for all our endeavors.

I also wish to acknowledge the kind patience of my children, who often pulled at my pants while I was at the computer, requesting "Papa, come and play with me."

About the Author

Dr Stephen Genuis practises Obstetrics and Gynecology in Alberta, Canada. He previously worked as a co-director of medical services in a hospital in rural Cameroon, West Africa. Currently, he serves as a board member on the Premier's Council in Support of Alberta Families as well as a committee member of the Physicians Continuing Care Committee for the College of Physicians and Surgeons of Alberta. His commitment to community education is evidenced by his many presentations to community groups, schools, and professional gatherings. His emphasis on education was acknowledged when he received the Resident of the Year Award from the University of Alberta graduating medical class of 1983. In 1991, Dr. Genuis was presented with a "Teacher of the Year Award" from the University of Alberta Department of Obstetrics and Gynecology.

KEG Publishing

Box 32025
#420, 2331-66 Street
Edmonton Alberta
Canada
T6K 4C2

(403) 461-1606

First Published in 1991
Second Edition 1992

Printed and Bound in Canada

Canadian Cataloguing in Publication Data
Genuis, Stephen J., 1955-
  Risky Sex
  1. Sexually transmitted diseases.   I. Title
RC200.G48 1991   616.95'1   C91-091106-1

ISBN # 0-9695080-0-X

I wish to thank a few people for their kind assistance, encouragement, suggestions and criticisms. Dr. Peter Petrik, Clinical Head of Pathology at Edmonton General Hospital, carefully scrutinized the material presented and made many invaluable suggestions; Dr. Shall Sinha kindly and skillfully directed my efforts with regards to publishing; Dr. Dieter W. Lemke provided many thoughtful recommendations for improvement; Muriel Lavin R.N. has provided endless vitality in promoting the material; Richard and Ursula Taylor, as non medical people, assured the readability of the book; Ronald Stephens and his committee of parents have provided much impetus on the need for such a manuscript; Holly Crowell's secretarial skills and assistance were appreciated; Vernie Wynnyk managed the day to day affairs of the book in a tireless and dedicated fashion.

Finally, I am grateful to my parents and siblings. Their encouragement and support are invaluable.

Contents

Introduction

As I sat to write the beginnings of this manuscript, I pondered and reflected on the meaning of books. Through the written word, people are able to vicariously live almost any experience imaginable. With our noses in a book, we are able to laugh, cry, love, hate, learn and relearn as we sit comfortably in one spot. Some works of literature are to educate, and some are to entertain. Books may be written to expose, others to malign, many to earn profit, and frequently books are used as a vehicle to communicate the ideas, thoughts and feelings of the author. By opening the cover of a book, we are able to escape to unfamiliar times and places again and again.

This piece is meant to educate and to provoke. The tragedy of Sexually Transmitted Diseases is not a vicarious problem and, unfortunately, our current world cannot escape from it. In my view, it is imperative to expose the problem so that adequate measures can be undertaken to deal with the current crisis. It is only in educating ourselves and others, and in facing the problem honestly and directly, that we can hope to overcome it.

Chapter #1

Why a Book on Sexually Transmitted Diseases?

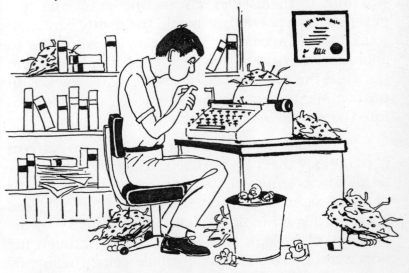

As I was preparing for my specialist exams in Obstetrics and Gynecology, I thought that I had read nearly everything that had been written in my field of medicine. I spent each late afternoon and evening studying the medical literature, reading about recent scientific findings, and analyzing clinical studies of patients. Then, as I drove my fiancee home from her University classes, I would rehearse aloud my answers for contrived examination questions. As the exam date neared, I felt satiated with information and, fortunately for my sake, my efforts were successful. However, despite my academic knowledge, I knew little about all the suffering and pain I would encounter daily in my medical practice.

When I started independent practice in Obstetrics and Gynecology seven years ago, I was absolutely amazed at the enormous power that was given to me by having an M.D. following my name. We live in a world where people usually keep their thoughts, feelings, and emotions to themselves, and yet patients, who had never seen me previously, would frequently bare their souls to me, a complete stranger. I have come to appreciate this special privilege, but have also come to recognize the awesome responsibility that follows. With the commencement of clinical practice, my education into the workings of the real world had begun.

I rarely saw much of the exotic details and patterns of pathology that I had studied so intensely just a few months before. Instead, I began to see recurrent patterns of stress, sadness, and loneliness that I had not read about in my gynecology books. As it turned out, the majority of patients that initially came through my door were teenagers and young single women frequently with unplanned pregnancies. About seventy per cent of my maternity case load in those first years of practice was unmarried women. These women faced many and diverse challenges and were often involved in very disturbing social situations.

After a short period of time it became increasingly clear that there was a huge menace in this population; a problem not as visible as unplanned pregnancy, yet far more prevalent. Day after day, I began to recognize the great numbers of patients who presented with Sexually Transmitted Diseases (STDs) or complications of these afflictions. At first, I thought perhaps this problem was confined to individuals from poor socio-economic backgrounds, but as my practice widened to include women from all creeds, colors, occupations, and backgrounds, it became apparent that this problem was ubiquitous, without discrimination, and it is getting worse.

The objective of this book is to clearly outline the current status of sexually transmitted diseases. Rather than focusing on detailed medical facts and trivia, which may be important to caregivers, I would like to emphasize the extent of the problem, the ramifications, and general strategies for dealing with the crisis. Finally, it is my hope that the information will not only assist the lay person in making personal decisions but will also equip individuals to respond to pertinent educational programs and political decisions in a cognizant and informed manner.

Chapter #2

How Often Do STDs Occur?

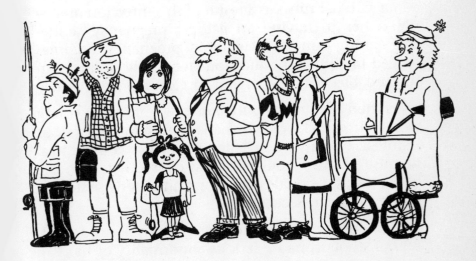

When assessing the incidence of Sexually Transmitted Diseases (STDs), it is important to include both the direct and indirect presentations of this problem. In other words, there are some people who come in with a concern that they have an STD and wish to have it diagnosed and treated; and others that have symptoms or medical complaints that result from complications of an STD. When trying to estimate how often these diseases occur, it is also important to remember that vast numbers of people are not aware of being infected and that many who are aware, may never seek help or assistance for their condition. This chapter will begin with some case studies to illustrate the variety of presentations often seen, followed by facts and figures detailing the extent of the problem.

One morning, I was urgently called into the hospital to see and operate on a woman who had a ruptured pregnancy in her fallopian tube. This frightened individual had previously contracted a pelvic infection, commonly known as Pelvic Inflammatory Disease, from a sexually acquired infection as a teenager. The damage to her tubes as a result of this infection predisposed her to having an ectopic pregnancy, a life-threatening condition where a pregnancy becomes lodged in the wrong location frequently resulting in rupture, bleeding and urgent surgical management.

I then went to my office and saw a pregnant young woman in early labor, who had just developed a serious outbreak of active herpes lesions in her genital area. Because of the serious potential consequences to the child, it was necessary to perform an otherwise unnecessary Cesarean Section.

The next patient, a fourteen year old junior-high school student, had a serious abnormality of her Pap smear indicating the pre-cancerous condition of her cervix. She had contacted a sexually transmitted virus called HPV (Human Papilloma Virus) after a brief encounter with a new partner. This virus has been identified to be an oncogenic(cancer causing) virus and was likely the cause of the serious problem that had developed in her cervix.

Shortly after that, a local physician working in the area of STDs called to discuss a teenage woman whom I had just delivered. The patient had tested positive for the AIDS virus and yet, regardless of the risks of transmission, was continuing to work as a prostitute . She refused any counselling and, in fact, refused to believe that she was carrying the virus despite repeated tests confirming that she was infected. Her child, now only a few weeks old, had been neglected and was accordingly apprehended by the child welfare department shortly after birth. Although the infant also tested positive for the AIDS virus, it is difficult to determine, for a number of months, whether this is just a reflection of his mother's infection markers still in his bloodstream, or whether he will indeed have the disease himself. He has about a thirty to fifty per cent chance of having AIDS and passing away in the first few years of his young life.

The next patients were a married couple who had been trying unsuccessfully to conceive a pregnancy over the last four years. After establishing that the husband's semen production was normal, and that the wife was ovulating normally, we elected to visualize her pelvic structures directly through a minor surgical procedure called a laparoscopy. As an adolescent, she had contracted an STD called Chlamydia and there was concern regarding the effect this infection may have had on her reproductive organs. Unfortunately, both of her fallopian tubes were blocked with excessive scarring and adhesions in her pelvis. It was a difficult task to relate the poor prognosis. As we discussed the slim chance of the woman conceiving a child naturally, it was heartbreaking to witness the tears of this young couple.

After seeing a couple of excited, expectant mothers for prenatal visits, I was confronted by an angry, recently divorced, middle aged woman, complaining bitterly of ongoing vaginal discharge and pelvic pain. She had acquired an STD sometime previously and, despite many treatments, she continued to complain of incapacitating discomfort she had never had prior to her infection.

These case studies are representative of the many victims of this ongoing scourge in our society. Despite the explosion in medical technologies, the incidence of these infections continues to escalate at an alarming rate. Although there is a small percentage of people who come to see health professionals directly expressing concern that they currently have a STD, there is a whole multitude of individuals who present to physicians offices, Emergency Departments at hospitals, and to public health clinics, complaining of symptoms and problems which are the direct or indirect consequence of STDs.

In the medical literature there appears to be ever increasing reports on the prevalence and complications associated with STDs. Many studies have been carried out to ascertain trends and to get an overall idea of what is happening in this area. The recent results are truly alarming.

In most major cities, there are STD clinics which have been established to provide screening and treatment for afflictions of this nature. The attendance at these centers has been increasing and each year about 5 million people are assessed at STD clinics throughout the United States.[1] In addition to this it seems that about equal numbers annually visit their private physicians with the same problems.[2]

A recent World Health Organization report indicated that one in twenty teenagers and young adults worldwide contract one form or another of STDs each year! A report from the American Social Health Association indicates that "about two people are infected every five seconds" in the United States and Canada.[3]

It is very difficult to determine the exact prevalence of each type of STD and many feel that the real extent of the problem is even worse than estimates of trends would suggest. When a person has a pregnancy, she generally presents to a physician or to a health care worker at some point regarding her pregnancy and her baby is usually delivered by a medical professional. The birth is recognized and a statistic, as well as a child, is born. Individuals with STDs, however, do not necessarily make themselves known. This may occur because many of these infections have no direct early symptoms and the individual infected, or their physician, may be unable to detect the presence of infection. Those who recognize that they are afflicted may not seek help and thus the problem at its early stages may not be identified.

Affected individuals may be afraid to be tested for certain types of infections because of fear that a positive result may label them and have negative repercussions for their life. In addition, many STDs are not "reportable". Reportable diseases require that physicians report the presence of these infections to a central agency which assimilates the data and produces figures and results. If the presence of certain STDs are not reported, it is very difficult to gather accurate information regarding their frequency.

These are some of the reasons why it is difficult to document the exact severity and extent of the problem. Let us now look at some specific diseases and what the medical literature suggests has been evolving from an epidemiologic perspective.

A study in the first four months of 1989 in Quebec approximated that one in every 394 women living in Montreal is infected with HIV! (Human Immunodeficiency Virus-the organism responsible for AIDS) and that in New York City, one in every 77 women is infected with this lethal virus.

Recent studies have estimated that somewhere between 26 and 31 million individuals in the U.S.A.are currently infected with genital herpes.[4] The genital herpes virus is the main cause of genital ulcers in North America and the total number of physician-patient visits to deal with this disease has gone up by 1500% between 1966 and 1987.[5] The incidence of this herpes infection reported in newborn children has increased by about 400% in many areas in the last twenty years.[6]

A recent submission by the Cancer Committee of the Society of Obstetricians and Gynecologists of Canada discussed the human papilloma virus and its relation to cancers in the female genital tract. They indicate that:

"It is now recognized that the human papilloma virus (HPV) are STD pathogens of major epidemiologic importance with a wider clinical spectrum and a higher epidemic incidence than previously suspected with approximately 20% of the female population between the ages of 15-40 harboring this virus." [7]

In the American Journal of Diseases of Children, a study recently reported the findings of the extent of HPV in the teenage population. Sexually active women, 13 to 21 years of age were tested for evidence of HPV infection at the time they went for a routine pap smear. Evidence of this virus was found in 38% of these young women, many of whom had had only a single partner! [8] The estimates for people presenting with complaints related to new infections with genital herpes and genital human papilloma virus, which represents only a portion of those that are actually carrying the disease, range up to one million new cases each year.[9][10]

The Centres for Disease Control in the United States estimates that 4 million new cases of chlamydial infection occur each and every year. A considerable number of these infections will lead to serious and permanent complications such as sterility and chronic pelvic scarring.

Many people in the general public are under the impression that some of the traditional STDs have disappeared. In reality, however, the incidence of some previously declining infections, has skyrocketed. For example, the rate of syphilis infection in the United States has been increasing since 1978 and is at its highest level in forty years.[11] The rate of this infection in newborn children, despite all the therapies that are available, is rising seriously. A study reviewing the rate change of newborn syphilis infection in New York between 1986 to 1988 indicates that the number of reported cases increased more than 500% in these two years.[12] A similar study in Miami showed a threefold increase over the same time period. [13]

There appears to be a number of co-factors associated with the increased prevalence of STDs. Studies indicate that there has been a significant correlation between illicit drug usage and the increasing incidence of certain types of STDs. One of the reasons is the increasing number of individuals exchanging sex for drugs.[14] The ever-present problem of alcohol abuse also appears to compound the problem, as intoxicated persons often have difficulty making informed and appropriate health decisions.

Rapid international travel has become yet another

factor in the dramatic spread of STDs. Whereas in the past we were more likely to see certain areas having outbreaks of infections, now, the whole world is placed at some degree of risk. The rapid spread of the AIDS virus is only one example of how many current STDs are spread by individuals travelling around the globe, both infecting and being infected by individuals of the host country.[15] Another example of this can be seen in the international spread of certain types of antibiotic-resistant gonorrhea.[16] The sprouting up of pockets of this organism in certain areas of the world point to the itinerary of the infecting agents.

Over the last few years, world attention has become focused on the AIDS virus and much of the concern pertains to the serious situation in some African nations. A number of years ago I had the pleasure of working in a small hospital in an African country and thus I have a keen interest as to the ongoing status of health care in this area of the world. A contact who has recently been doing research on the prevalence of some infectious diseases in a particular African nation has very disturbing stories to tell. She indicated that one hundred per cent of the prostitutes she tested were positive for the AIDS virus in the capital city of this country. Furthermore, about seventy per cent of the female population she tested in this region were also positive for this same virus. She claimed that the official statistics released by the country reflected only a fraction of the real number, as high rates might be detrimental to the tourist trade, a very important part of the country's economy. Finally, she was 'encouraged' to leave the country when the full purpose of her visit was discovered.

Anecdotal tales relate how some African villages

have only elderly people and young children remaining and even news reports are beginning to announce the extent of the tragedy in this continent. Under the headline "AIDS may soon engulf all of Africa", a recent newspaper article related that "In one Tanzanian village, one in every five people have died from the disease." [17] An interview with the head of the AIDS unit for an international development agency, reported in the Medical Post " I've been to villages where there are more graves than houses, and there are grandparents looking after a lot of kids." She further relates "I can tell you all kinds of stories about mortuaries overloaded , and people so tired of burying people that they can hardly do it properly anymore...".[18] It now appears that AIDS is the leading cause of death in most central African cities. We North Americans, however, cannot forget that we now live in a global village. AIDS has become the leading cause of death for women aged 20-40 in major cities in the Americas and Western Europe. [19]

To sum up, the current problem of STDs is escalating, it is worldwide, it is nondiscriminating to color, age, or sexual preference, and there is no consistent evidence that this upward spiralling trend is levelling off.

Chapter #3

Which Are the Common STDs?

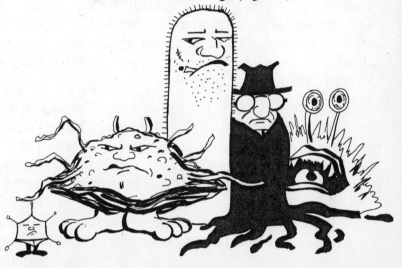

I recently had the pleasure of speaking at a local school to a group of Junior High School students on the topic of STDs. After the session was over, a young adolescent boy sheepishly inquired "If you give an STD to your partner, you get rid of it yourself, don't you?" Although the question may sound humorous, it certainly illustrates the need for a clear understanding of the ramifications and significance of various STDs. In order to have this clear understanding, however, one must acquire a basic knowledge of what the common diseases are, and recognize some of the particular idiosyncrasies peculiar to each infective agent. And to answer the student's question: No, the infecting organisms enter, invade and inhabit the new host, but also remain an integral part of the old host.

A variety of expressions have been, and are being used to describe infections caught by having sexual relations with an infected partner. The vernacular has included such terms as venereal diseases, "the dose", "clap", "V.D.", and many other colorful terms and phrases. The term Sexually Transmitted Diseases, or STDs, as they are affectionately known, is the current umbrella term which encompasses afflictions for which sexual contact is an important, though not necessarily the only, avenue of acquisition.

There are different groups of infective organisms which have the potential to cause illness. Some of the more common categories are Bacteria, Viruses, Protozoa, Parasites, and Fungi. Each group of organisms has particular characteristics and it is important to distinguish between them as certain treatments can be effective against one type of organism but not against the others. For example, antibiotics are very efficient at treating certain types of bacterial infections, but these potentially lifesaving and miraculous drugs are usually ineffective against viral infections. This is clearly illustrated in the case of the common cold, a malady usually caused by a virus. The use of antibiotics in an effort to cure the viral cold frequently results in frustration and possibly even side effects from the drug itself.

There are many infections which may be passed by sexual contact and which have the potential to cause serious damage. However, I would like to give a brief overview of six common organisms and one common clinical presentation that account for the overwhelming majority of the STDs that we are currently witnessing. These common STDs have been chosen for discussion as they permit the illustration of some of the concerns and principles that need emphasis. A more detailed and comprehensive study of these and other STDs may be found in other excellent reference books. We will discuss Gonorrhea, Chlamydia, and Syphilis from the bacterial contingent; Genital Herpes, Human Papilloma Virus, and the AIDS virus (HIV) from the viral section; and mention will be made of a condition called Non-Gonococcal Urethritis (NGU) in males and its counterpart Muco-Purulent Cervicitis (MPC) in women.

GONORRHEA

Gonorrhea is caused by a bacterial organism known as Neisseria gonorrheae. It can have many sites of infection but most commonly it affects the cervix in women and the anterior portion of the urethra in men. The rectal area, the throat, and the eyes are also potential sites of infection in both sexes and, if untreated, the organism can potentially spread to different areas in the body.

Men may complain of burning discomfort when they urinate and may also notice a discharge of pus from the end of their penis. Although the majority of men who are infected recognize some symptoms, it is felt that about twenty per cent have no complaints and carry the bacteria silently. When the organism is carried in the throat, there are usually no symptoms at all. Without medical attention, this organism can spread to infect the man's prostate or testicles and may be transmitted to sexual partners.

The infection is particularly insidious in females as about eighty per cent of women have no symptoms in the early stages of the infection. There may be some vaginal discharge or some discomfort when urinating.

If the infection is unrecognized, as is often the case, the organism frequently spreads to infect the uterus and the fallopian tubes and may result in sterility.

In children, there are two types of infection. The eyes of a newborn may be infected as a result of acquiring the disease at or during birth with the potential to cause serious damage and even blindness. In addition, a young boy or girl may be afflicted with this bacteria as a victim of direct sexual contact from another individual carrying the organism.

When the illness is recognized and then treated with appropriate antibiotic agents, the infecting organism that causes gonorrhea usually is eradicated effectively. However, damage caused by the organism is not usually reversed once the acute infection is treated.

CHLAMYDIA

Over the last few years, chlamydia has been recognized as one of the most prevalent and most damaging sexually transmitted infections. The organism, Chlamydia trachomatis, is a type of bacterium which grows within living cells. Much research in the last few years has allowed easier recognition and treatment.

The manifestations of this problem vary between the sexes. In the man, chlamydial infection is often without symptoms, although about half of the men infected have some complaints. Common presentations of this illness include pain on urination, discharge from the tip of the penis, or an altered or itchy sensation at the end of the penile area.

Chlamydia, like some other STDs, appears to be sexist in nature in that women bear a disproportionate incidence of complications and consequences. Once again, the vast majority of women carrying this infection have no symptoms at early stages of the infective process. Even in the absence of any noticeable symptoms, damage of the female reproductive organs may progress to result in a variety of serious complications.

The newborn child is also a potential victim of this kind of infection. The predominant sites of infection are the eyes and the lungs. Chlamydia may cause corneal scarring and visual impairment if left untreated, and also has the potential to cause pneumonia.

There are now effective and easily available tests to diagnose this condition if the infected individual or their physician suspects a problem. Although therapy with appropriate antibiotics usually eliminates these bacteria, there is frequently significant residual damage if the infection is not treated in the early stages.

SYPHILIS

This particular organism has a long and sordid past, having infected and destroyed many famous individuals over the centuries. It is thought by many that this disease is a thing of the past, but this sinister germ is in the process of making a resurgence, including a profound escalation in the newborn population.

Syphilis is caused by an organism called Treponema pallidum, and is transmitted by direct contact with an infected sore. If left untreated, the disease passes through a series of phases. About three weeks after the initial contact, the new recipient develops a painless lesion in the genital area, the hallmark of Primary Syphilis. This lesion spontaneously heals in a few weeks and is followed by the appearance of numerous skin lesions and a flu-like illness about six weeks later. This stage subsides in about three weeks and the disease enters the Latent Stage. At this point, there are generally no significant complaints or noticeable changes noted by the victim.

Following this latent phase, the disease appears to have a variable course if left untreated. The process may remain in the latent phase with intermittent relapses similar to secondary syphilis; the infection has been reported to be spontaneously cured in some fortunate individuals; or the illness may proceed to tertiary syphilis which may affect various organs in the body including the brain, the heart, the bones and other sites.

The infection appears to be most contagious during the Primary, Secondary, and early Latent phases of the illness. But one of the most serious tragedies in our current world is the increase in the rates of congenital syphilis—when a newborn child has been infected while developing in the mother's uterus prior to birth. The child may pass away, or may have a variety of serious defects, including central nervous system abnormalities and bone alterations.

Antibiotic therapies remain extremely effective in treating and eliminating the infecting agent from the human system. Appropriate therapy is determined by the site and stage of infection but the complications and damage caused by syphilis may persist even after treatment.

HUMAN PAPILLOMA VIRUS (HPV)

In the last few years, it has become increasingly evident that HPV is a sexually transmitted infection of major proportion and with serious ramifications.

This virus had previously been recognized to cause genital warts (known in the medical world as condylomata accuminata) in a minority of individuals infected with this virus. These small, painless growths, found in the genital area, pose a nuisance as they are sometimes hard to eradicate and often spread quickly. Even after initial removal of the growths, the virus itself still remains present, with the potential to cause recurrent warts. These fleshy, cauliflower lesions may be found in many sites in the genital area including the penis, scrotum, and anus in men. In women, common sites include the vagina, vulva, clitoris, and anus. The virus has also been isolated from the oral cavity in adults and has been associated with small growths on the vocal cords of children who may have contacted the infecting organism at birth.

As with many of the other STDs, this viral infection is often without symptoms in the early stages and was previously considered by many to be of minimal concern. However, recent evidence strongly suggests that HPV may cause precancerous and cancerous changes of certain areas of the female genital tract. This accounts for the serious increase in the incidence of cervical cancer in the last decade. There is also suspicion that it may cause cancer in other sites in the body and current research is beginning to shed more light in this direction. In addition, HPV infection is associated with impaired healing of the perineum after childbirth (the perineum is the area of skin below the outer vagina which may require healing after the birth process). [1] Some medical professionals have labelled HPV as the "STD of the 1990s". Yet, it has received little attention as it is overshadowed by the more lethal AIDS virus.

The HPV infection is highly contagious and appears to spread easily upon sexual contact. There is at least a 50% chance of transmission with a single sexual encounter with an infected person.[2] Once acquired, there is no current method of eliminating it. Although the usual avenue of spreading this virus is by sexual relations, it is believed that transmission by certain objects such as toilet seats and towels is possible.[3]

GENITAL HERPES - HERPES SIMPLEX VIRUS (HSV)

Herpes simplex virus appears to cause infection by direct contact from a sore of an infected person to the skin of the recipient, often during sexual contact. Newly infected individuals will often develop a first episode or outbreak of herpes. Initial attacks vary in intensity but frequently involve a cluster of painful sores or ulcers which may last for up to three weeks prior to healing. During this time, the virus migrates up the nerve fibres where it often remains dormant for varying lengths of time.

The infected individual may then develop recurrent attacks for the remainder of his or her life. In these recurrent episodes, the sores typically last for up to a week after which they usually clear up and the virus returns to a dormant stage. Available antiviral therapies appear to shorten the outbreaks, and when taken on a chronic basis, certain drugs may diminish the frequency of recurrences. However, the disease cannot be cured in that there are no means to destroy and eradicate the virus from the infected person.

When this disease is contacted by a newborn, it has a devastating potential for death or serious neurologic consequences.

AIDS - HUMAN IMMUNODEFICIENCY VIRUS (HIV)

HIV, Human Immunodeficiency Virus, is the accepted name designated to the virus, or viruses, that are responsible for causing Acquired Immunodeficiency Syndrome, commonly known as AIDS. HIV is a type of virus, referred to as a Retrovirus , which has the special ability to invade the normal cells of the infected individual, and to command these normal cells to become HIV producing cells.

These viruses have a particular attraction to certain cells which are part of the immune system, the mechanism within the body that is normally responsible for preventing and defending against infection and cancerous growths. With time, the normal cells are destroyed and lose their indispensable ability to protect the individual, thus leaving the person vulnerable to serious infections, tumor formation, and eventually to death.

AIDS refers to a condition found when HIV infected persons suffer from a variety of infections or cancerous complications secondary to a deficient immune system. After initially acquiring the AIDS virus, the vast majority of infected people feel perfectly well and often have no awareness of their infected state or no insight into the fact that they are infectious to others. It is not fully understood why some infected individuals develop fully expressed AIDS shortly after contacting the AIDS virus, and why others seem to carry the virus for a considerable length of time before developing serious symptoms. There appear to be some additional factors, or other influences which may come to bear on the rapidity of disease expression. From various epidemiologic studies, it appears that in adults the average time from the initial HIV infection to development of AIDS is 7-10 years.[4] In very young children, the development of full blown AIDS often occurs within two years of infection with the virus.

NON-GONOCCOCAL URETHRITIS

Many STDs can be delineated and diagnosed according to the infecting organism. However, health professionals frequently encounter patients complaining of a specific set of symptoms that, as a set, have become somewhat recognizable and given medical titles.

A frequent complaint heard in physicians offices from male patients is that of burning discomfort on urination. The patient may also complain of an associated discharge from the end of his penis. This condition is often suggestive of urethritis. This type of infection, often sexually transmitted, may be caused by Chlamydia or gonorrhea, but it is sometimes caused by organisms which cannot be identified and thus enters the category of a so-called non-gonococcal urethritis.

Similarly, in the female, complaints of abnormal vaginal discharge, or irregular spotting may sometimes point to an inflammation of the cervix. This alteration of the cervix may be attributable to an infection by a variety of organisms, including chlamydia, herpes, gonorrhea and others. This presentation in the female patient may be described as muco-purulent cervicitis.

Chapter #4

Where are the Experts and What Do Their Statistics Show?

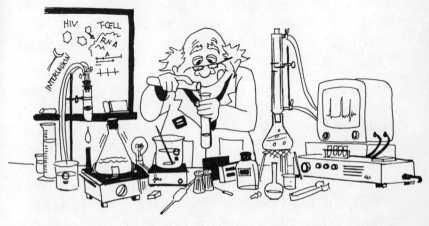

At an early stage in my training, I had the opportunity to observe a scientist who was heavily involved in research. He was well known for being an expert and an authority in one specific area. He was the author of many papers as well as sections in books, and frequently gave talks and workshops about his area of expertise. He was very articulate and came across as an entertaining and delightful speaker.

The research technicians and I observed that some of the techniques used, as well as the interpretation of the findings, were very questionable. I began to realize that conclusions and recommendations that are derived from studies may be based on subjective testing or biased interpretation, and thus reflect the perspective of the reseacher. It was at this point that I began to question the previously blind acceptance of information, statistics and counsel from so-called experts.

Although there is an abundance of invaluable study and research that goes on every day, it is crucial that the readers carefully analyze and question the process prior to accepting the results and conclusions. With particular reference to the social sciences, which often do not have black and white results, I have sometimes observed contradictory conclusions from the same data.

In light of these types of experiences, I have become very careful when I read or hear the results of studies. All too often these days, I hear someone say, "Recent studies have shown..." or "It has been definitively proven in studies that...". An example that comes to mind is found in some authoritative comments I once heard from opposing sides on the divisive abortion debate. When discussing the aftermath of abortion, I heard an articulate woman relate that studies have proven conclusively that there is no such thing as post abortion trauma. She stated that a recent study showed 99.8% of women were relieved to have had their abortion. I was particularly struck when a speaker from the other side of this difficult debate indicated that recent studies had shown that 96% of women regretted having their abortion and had been pressured into it rather than choosing it themselves. After reading contradictory statistics in various studies over and over again in the last few years, I have come to agree with the phrase that 'Statistics conceal more than they reveal'. The famous Mark Twain quotation states: "There are lies, damn lies, and statistics."

A most notable example in this area relates to unplanned pregnancy in various provinces in Canada. In one province, there had been much criticism of the local government for the high rate of teenage pregnancy when compared to certain other provinces. Newspaper articles and various reports and individuals quoted statistics lambasting current programs aimed at preventing unwed pregnancy. Many politicians appeared to respond to the criticism and efforts were addressed to correct this seeming disparity in pregnancy rates. Having both an interest and much experience in this area, I carefully reviewed the publications and the statistics quoted. It became apparent that the major difference in rates could be explained by the fact that the provinces with the lower rates had free standing abortion clinics where terminated pregnancies were not reported and thus not included in the rates for unwanted pregnancies.

I also recently heard a statistic that 74% of mothers were now in the work force and thus politicians should face up to this current reality and design and fund programs to meet the need of the majority. On closer examination, however, this 74% included those that earned any income at all, whether it be teaching gymnastics for two hours each week, doing accounting in the evening at home, or selling crafts at Christmas bazaars.

The list of examples of misleading statistics goes on ad infinitum, but suffice it to say that it is important once again to research and investigate before believing. We are currently living in a world of experts and authorities from whose lips ebulliently flow unending facts and figures. One only has to listen to newscasts or documentaries to hear these sagacious individuals pontificate about everything and anything.

While listening to our national radio station on my drives to and from the hospital, I have listened to authorities on parenting, education, playing, economics, self-esteem, family, politics, women's issues and more. There appears to be an 'authority mentality' affecting our society. All too often I hear from patients that they followed one path of action for their life because of what they read or heard from some expert. Some individuals, unfortunately, leave behind their own instincts and common sense because of direction that has been given to them from a so-called authority.

One only has to listen to two expert economists, both with scintillating degrees, argue eloquently in contradictory fashions about the direction of the economy. Or consider a panel of so-called political experts from opposing parties who interpret events and government decisions reaching contradictory conclusions. How can this be if they are all experts? When viewing this scenario it is imperative to look at the agenda or motivation behind the conclusions reached. In other words, why is the individual saying what he or she is saying?

I recently had the opportunity to attend a lecture series featuring a world renowned physician and author. I was looking forward to meeting him as I had repeatedly read and studied his textbook in preparation for my specialist exams. He was discussing some of his research and honestly stated that when doing studies, "...people have an agenda that they are trying to prove." He went on to caution his audience that when reading the findings and conclusions, it is important to take into consideration "who is writing it and what is the prejudice that they are going into the study with."[1]

In the area of STDs, it is equally important that individuals and groups challenge the information that is being directed at them by experts, authorities, and those reporting the information. In 1983, for example, people read that AIDS was a 'gay plague', transmitted only by homosexual acts. At that time, many people accepted this assumption and continued or became involved in a lifestyle that placed them at risk for AIDS. This gravely erroneous message, that AIDS is a 'gay disease', unfortunately seems to have remained in the minds of huge numbers in the general public. I recall listening to a presentation by a researcher who was billed as an expert on AIDS. He related on the airwaves how it had been conclusively demonstrated that it was extremely hard to catch AIDS and it was transmitted solely by high risk sexual activities and exchange of blood. Five years later, it has been shown to be transmitted by breast feeding, transmitted to a child during pregnancy, transmitted through skin sores exposed to the virus, and potentially passed on by other routes as well.

In the early 1980s, I also heard repeatedly from authorities on AIDS that only 10% of those infected with the virus would develop the disease. The assurance was given that 90% of those infected would live a full life unhampered by the devastation of the AIDS syndrome. It is now the opinion of many researchers that most, if not all those infected with the virus, will eventually be afflicted with this disease.

I have heard some experts recently claim that the severity of the AIDS epidemic has been grossly overstated.

It has been suggested that the number of newly positive HIV tests are lower than had been anticipated and that the recent statistics on the number of positive tests suggests that the AIDS problem is in fact, diminishing. In response, I would like to summarize a conversation I recently had with an intelligent, capable and experienced physician who has been directly involved with caring for many HIV infected persons.

We discussed the concerns that health care workers share regarding the risks of contacting HIV. Our conversation included discussion of a recent article in the "AIDS ALERT" publication which related that an HIV infected gynecologist was "forced out of a medical partnership despite his offer to do no 'hands on' work"[2], and that a similarly infected "director of anesthesiology was denied contact with patients and then disciplined when he assisted a patient who had vomited and was in immediate danger of aspirating"[3], a situation that may have resulted in serious illness or death for the patient if assistance had not been provided. When I asked my colleague her views on regular HIV testing for physicians because of the potential risks of transmitting infection to patients, she replied that she had considered the outcome of a positive test result in herself. She hypothesized that if she was infected and this fact became known, her medical practice could potentially be altered: patients may be afraid to come to her for medical care, some of her colleagues may shun her, and her situation as the sole breadwinner in her family would be threatened. This physician felt that it is quite understandable why increasing numbers of people sense that they have much to lose and little to gain by being tested for HIV.

It is becoming apparent that many known HIV infected patients are unfortunately being ostracized, rejected, and scorned, and so it is no wonder that increasing numbers of individuals are reluctant to have HIV testing. Accordingly, if many of the people at potential risk are not being tested repeatedly, it is difficult to provide accurate figures and statistics. The claim that the AIDS problem is diminishing simply because of a decrease in the reported numbers of HIV positive tests in a few centers is disturbing and misleading. In fact, according to the Surveillance Report by the Centers for Disease Control, the overall rate of increase in the new cases of active AIDS in the United States went from 9 percent in 1989 to 23 percent in 1990.[4]

There are many other examples where so-called authorities have made dogmatic statements about enigmatic STDs and have later been shown to be clearly in the wrong. The problem, of course, with making such bold claims is that people live their lives and make decisions about their sexuality based on the information presented to them. I feel it is counterproductive to present uncertain information as reality and fact to the unsuspecting lay population. It is equally deceiving and counterproductive to portray optimism and false hope simply to allay anxiety and concern, when it is often this same anxiety and concern that finally demands and heralds change and action.

Yet, there have also been some who appear to have overstated or exaggerated the seriousness of the problem. In 1986, I read a book devoted to the problem of AIDS which suggested that there would be about 64 million American persons infected with AIDS by the end of 1990. In 1987, another source claimed that 20% of heterosexuals would be dead from AIDS by the end of 1990. Although such scenarios may raise awareness of the problem of STDs, when reality does not fulfill such assessments, people may not heed or attend to any further claims stating the genuine status of the problem. Furthermore, individuals and groups who express valid concern may be lumped together with alarmists and doomsayers and thus be ignored.

There is much left to be discovered about the many STDs that are affecting our world. Before long, there will be new tests and new treatments; further consequences and methods of transmission may be recognized; and other organisms, not yet discovered or fully understood, may be found to be acting in association with known STD agents. Accordingly, it is likely that within a short time, some of the information in this book and other books in this field will be incomplete. But this is the nature of science and research. Until we are certain about the facts pertaining to STDs, we should be implementing strategies and precautions to address the most serious possibilities rather than making optimistic assumptions and living accordingly.

It is also noteworthy to remember that just as war and instability may result in clear profits to some individuals, the STD crisis also has raised profits for some organizations. Among the many periodicals and journals that arrive at my office is a free information pamphlet that comes on a quarterly basis. The stated intention is "Expanding Information and Improving Understanding about Reproductive Health and the Prevention of Sexually Transmitted Disease and Unplanned Pregnancy."[5] This literature is published under an educational grant from a major condom company. A solution to the AIDS crisis is offered on the front cover of the Summer 1987 edition "All that remains to be done is to get people to use condoms—properly..."[6]

My objective in this section is certainly not to diminish trust or to weaken faith in authority but rather to encourage individuals to be increasingly diligent in researching information which may impact on their lives. There is a considerable amount of conflicting information and misleading ideas that are being presented to the public today. The reasons for this vary from misunderstanding of statistics, through deliberate attempts to influence people, perhaps for political, economic, or other gain. It is important that people accept personal responsibility for their decisions and for the information they choose to believe.

By the same token, I invite the reader to question the information that I present in this book. It is not my main intent to impart knowledge or to suggest that I am an expert at anything. Rather, my objective is to encourage the reader to assess the current situation, research the available information, and to draw conclusions as he or she sees fit.

Chapter 5

How Do We Recognize an STD?

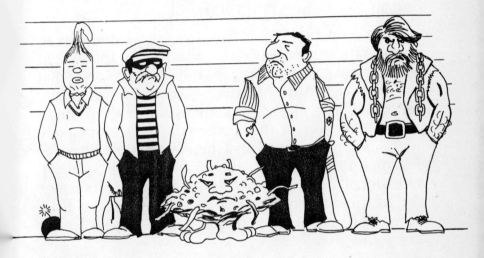

A few months ago, I had the pleasure of meeting a robust, energetic, athletic woman in her early twenties who presented to my office for a general gynecologic check. She indicated to me that finally she had met Mr. Right, a wonderful new male acquaintance, and was soon going to embark on a sexual relationship with him. Before commencing this relationship, however, she wished to make sure that she was "clean". In other words, she wanted to ensure that she wasn't carrying any disease or infection that she might pass on to her knight in shining armour.

I have heard this theme, and numerous variations of it, on many occasions. I have often had young women inquire if there is any way to detect the presence of STDs and some have wished to have their partners "checked out". Most commonly, patients have heard that if they suspect they have an infection or have been exposed to one, they should go to their doctor to be checked and treated. It is as if they think that there is a STD blood test that will determine the existence of any and all infections. Sadly, this is not the case.

For some types of STDs, there are reliable tests to confirm the existence of an organism in the individual. The presence of gonorrhea, syphilis and chlamydial infection can usually be diagnosed when specifically tested for. The major problem with the above mentioned infections is that patients may be completely without symptoms and may therefore never present for testing until significant complications have occurred. Occasionally, individuals will present to their physicians for treatment because they have been alerted by a sexual partner or by a public health official to the possibility of infection.

The presence of genital herpes can be confirmed by laboratory tests if the patient has active sores. When the disease enters its dormant stage, however, it is difficult or impossible for lab tests to confirm that the patient has this type of genital infection.

For patients who do not have any initial symptoms, such as genital warts, there are no reliable and easily accessible tests thus far for the human papilloma virus (HPV). However, under certain circumstances it can sometimes be identified by special techniques. Regardless of whether the virus is identified or not, the damage and destruction to the patient as well as the spread of the virus goes on. It is important to recall that the vast majority of patients have no discernible symptoms in the early stages of HPV infection.

Finally, the tests currently in widespread use to identify those with the AIDS infection, leave much to be desired. The tests measure a specific response to the virus rather than determining the actual presence of the virus. As a result, individuals may be infected by, and may transmit the virus for some time before its presence is confirmed by test results. As the recognition of HIV infection has some unique features with significant ramifications to many, it is important to discuss the diagnostic concerns with this illness.

A few months ago, a married, 28 year old teacher presented to the emergency department in a state of panic. She had been married for four years and had finally, after eighteen months, conceived a pregnancy. She was currently about 11 weeks along and, until that evening, had been ecstatic and exuberant about the prospect of the new addition. That evening after supper, her husband appeared somewhat despondent and confessed that he was bisexual. He had just been informed that he had tested positive for HIV. She became terrified about how this might affect the baby and came to the Emergency Department hoping to have her questions answered. First, she wished to know if she was infected; secondly, she wished to know what the chances would be of the baby being infected; thirdly, she wished to know the ultimate outcome to the child if the infant was infected; and so on.

It was explained to this patient that we do not have a readily available test to determine the presence of the AIDS virus. Instead, the currently available testing procedure looks for a reaction to the virus. This reaction is called an antibody and may be found in the infected individual's bloodstream. The test, therefore, identifies the antibody rather than the virus itself. This reaction to the virus and development of antibodies occurs after a variable length of time, anywhere from a few weeks to many years. Thus a person may be infected with the virus, with the ability to transmit this virus to another individual or to a developing child, and yet may test completely negative to the antibody test. If the antibody test is confirmed positive, then one can be reasonably certain that the individual has been infected; if the test is negative, it is not determined whether or not the individual is afflicted. This particular woman tested negative and thus may or may not be infected. If infected with the virus, despite the absence of antibodies and negative test results, many estimate that between 30-50% of subsequent offspring will be infected by the time of birth. Some recent research, however, has suggested that the rate of transmission from mother to child may be lower than previously anticipated.[1] Many of the afflicted children will die within two years.

Although many experts dogmatically believe otherwise, it has now been established beyond a doubt that there are numerous people who will carry the virus for many years, while their AIDS antibody test remains negative.[2] In a recent publication of the well respected New England Journal of Medicine, a long term study reported on a number of men known to be carrying the AIDS virus. The overwhelming majority of participants continued to test negative, with the commonly performed AIDS antibody test, for more than three years after contacting the infection.[3] Accordingly, it is difficult to have an accurate idea of how many people, and which people are infected with this lethal virus.

Furthermore, many of the people who now have AIDS contacted the disease prior to the time when the illness was even discovered. With a latency period of up to 10 years or more before infected people show signs of illness[4], it will be another number of years before we know how many people are currently infected. Tragically, the greater the number of individuals who are infected with HIV, the greater the rate of spread as the potential sources of infection exponentially escalate. As reported in the Journal of the American Medical Association

As the prevalence of infection in the population increases, the likelihood of infection in a random partner also increases. Therefore, in an epidemic, one would also expect to observe an increasing risk of infection as the prevalence of the infection increases.[5]

In the case of both AIDS and other STDs, I have heard the comment that "he's not that sort of guy" or that he is "real straight laced and clean cut" and thus could never be carrying an STD. Some people feel that those infected have a particular appearance, demeanor, or way of walking that might alert an observer to the presence of infection. As has been previously discussed, many of the common STDs have no symptoms in their early stages, and thus the patients do not notice any changes and will not have any complaints. They then pass them on to their contacts without ever knowing that they have an infection themselves. Accordingly, if the infected person is not aware of the presence of infection, it is hardly likely that a partner will be able to diagnose or anticipate the risk. For example, asymptomatic transmission of Herpes has become increasingly recognized in the last few years. Seventy-five per cent of persons who have been the source of infection for patients with diagnosed and documented

Herpes infection, denied any sores or evidence of infection at the time of contact and presumed transmission. (6, 7, 8)

In recent months, there has been the proliferation of commercial ventures offering individuals some sort of identification to display freedom from STDs to prospective sexual partners. Attempts are being made to obtain medical signatures on these documents to provide credibility to the owner of such material. There have also been clubs and groups that require freedom from STDs as a prerequisite for membership. With the inability to diagnose many of these infections, and with the ever changing status of each individual as he or she has relations, the false security that may be derived from these cards and these clubs is evident.

Finally, it is truly unfortunate that many members of the public have the mistaken notion that people with STDs generally belong to an identifiable or specific group. They may feel that certain STDs are confined to persons with specific sexual preferences or certain lifestyle habits such as drug abuse or prostitution. They may then falsely conclude that by avoiding contact with these specified groups or types of persons, that freedom from the risk of contacting STDs will be achieved. The situation with STDs, however, is much more involved than most people imagine. These viruses and bacteria do not appear to have race or lifestyle prejudices and are keen to become intimately involved with anyone who makes their acquaintance.

There is a new technology on the horizon, called PCR or polymerase chain reaction, which may revolutionize the ability to diagnose certain infections. This testing procedure is not available at this time for generalized commercial use as it is expensive, tedious, and susceptible to contamination. However, many predict that in the next few years, this test will be commonly used. Among the many potential uses of this advance, PCR analysis testing will be able to identify individuals infected with the AIDS virus without waiting for the development of antibodies, and will also be able to detect the presence of HPV. It may also serve to verify that transplanted organs and fluid donations, such as blood, are clearly free from transmissible infection. In addition, this test will potentially allow health officials to better assess the real prevalence of certain types of infection.

In conclusion, definitively recognizing some STDs is often difficult and frequently impossible. It is indeed a challenging situation when infected people may not know if they are carrying a disease of this type, when potential contacts have no way of identifying who may be infected, and when the medical profession is unable to diagnose many who are involved. It is tragic that many of these agents, travelling in a clandestine fashion, continue to maliciously ravage the afflicted individual and silently spread to unsuspecting contacts!

Chapter #6

How Do We Get Rid of an STD?

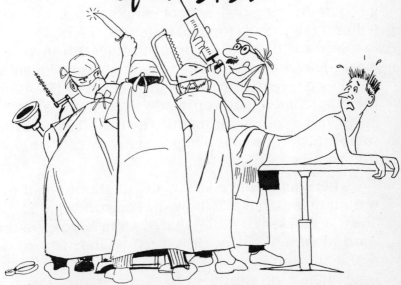

Most patients who see a physician or visit a clinic for assessment and treatment of STDs are under the impression that these illnesses can, for the most part, be treated and cured with antibiotic therapy. While this may be the case for STDs caused by bacteria, it is certainly not true for the viral infections.

With the modern day antibiotics that are available, gonorrhea, syphilis, and chlamydial infection can be effectively treated once they are suspected and diagnosed. Although the infecting organism may be eradicated, any damage occurring prior to treatment is not usually reversible. Serious complications, such as infertility, may require ongoing medical attention for years to come. It is thus very important for individuals who suspect they may be infected to seek medical attention as soon as possible. However, the increasingly ubiquitous viral STDs, including herpes, AIDS and genital warts, are not curable thus far.

I recently had occasion to see a fourteen year old girl, just entering high school, who had met a young fellow on the school football team. She quickly became involved and then, to her disappointment, disinvolved when he met another new student. She subsequently developed extensive genital warts (caused by HPV) and many attempts had been made to treat the affected areas with a topical ointment. The treatment was unsuccessful and she was referred to my care for surgical intervention.

This young lady asked many questions about the warts and inquired as to how she had contacted them. She was shocked to realize that, despite removal of the warts themselves, the virus persists and may cause repeated recurrences of these growths. At the present time, there is no treatment to eliminate the virus and once infected, a person continues to carry the virus indefinitely. She asked about spreading it to others, and I explained that the virus is transmitted by skin to skin contact. This bright young lady quickly concluded that she would likely pass this on to any subsequent sexual contact, "even a future husband" despite the use of condoms. Her spontaneous plea, "can't I even have a second chance?" was particularly moving as this adolescent had never previously heard of warts, let alone imagined that she may be afflicted with them indefinitely as a result of one sexual contact. It is indeed sad to reveal to any individual that they are infected with an incurable virus that they may readily pass on to other sexual contacts, as well as the possible spread to offspring.

Although there is no cure for viral STDs, there are two main avenues that have and are being explored in hopes of diminishing the prevalence and the severity of these afflictions. These are the development of immunizations to provide the body with a defense mechanism against the diseases themselves, and secondly, the use of certain drugs to diminish or delay the effect that the infection is having on the body.

The most publicized disease being researched with the goal of finding a vaccine and drugs for treatment is, of course, AIDS. There has been great hope that a vaccine will be developed to prevent any further spread of the Human Immunodeficiency Virus. While the objective of discovering a primary measure aimed at preventing rather than treating this disease is important, a sobering look at reality makes it hard to be too optimistic thus far. First of all, if a vaccine was found today, and appropriately distributed, there are already millions of people infected whose HIV status would not be reversed by vaccination. As far as I know, there is no vaccine available or close to being developed that has shown significant promise as a preventative measure against HIV. Secondly, the AIDS virus has already been found to have mutated, that is, to have changed slightly to form a second virus known as HIV-2. This nasty variation appears to have the same devastating potential as HIV-1, but a vaccine successful at preventing the first virus may not be successful against the second, mutated virus. Unfortunately the possibility remains that the virus may mutate yet again, to form other viruses with similar potential. At this time, there is some encouraging preliminary work suggesting that, perhaps at some point in the future, a vaccine may be developed that might slow down or theoretically halt the progression from HIV infection to the development of full blown AIDS.

I have often heard it expressed that it will not be long before effective drugs are found to turn AIDS into a chronic disease rather than a lethal one as it is now. AZT is an example of a drug currently being studied to determine its potential in this area. It has been shown to be extremely useful and beneficial to some infected individuals but, once again, there are concerns. First of all, these powerful agents often have very serious side effects which make it difficult for many individuals to tolerate taking them. When given to infected, but still asymptomatic individuals to delay onset of this disease, a seemingly healthy individual may become quite ill as a result of the medication. Secondly, these drugs are usually very expensive, and as the number of infected individuals continues to rise, the costs for use of these drugs, especially long term, will be astronomical. One can hope that effective antiviral agents capable of curing viral illness will be discovered and made available in the near future, but to my knowledge, there is no serious optimism in this regard.

It is indeed a frightening prospect to put together a composite picture of some of the points discussed regarding STDs. Many people do not know that they are carrying a sexually transmitted disease because they have no symptoms. Even if they suspect a problem, many of these diseases cannot be detected with the current testing techniques. Accordingly, these infections are spread unknowingly to sexual contacts who themselves commence another cycle of transmission. If diagnosed, many STDs have no cure and even if antibiotic treatment is possible, the physical complications may be lifelong. The ramifications to self, to partner and to offspring are very concerning. With this sobering scenario in mind, one cannot help but conclude that it is indeed time to begin to curb this escalating problem by stepping in before the cycle begins.

The sexual revolution of the last few decades has had a paradoxical effect. With the illusion of liberating people from repressive attitudes and lifestyles, many now suffer the bondage of lifelong sexually transmitted diseases or their consequences, from which there may be no liberation. It is interesting that Masters and Johnson, whose research and publications have had a tremendous impact on the sexual behaviour of many people, have commented that "...the sexual revolution is not yet dead—it's just that some of the troops are dying."[1]

Chapter #7

Are There Any Serious Complications?

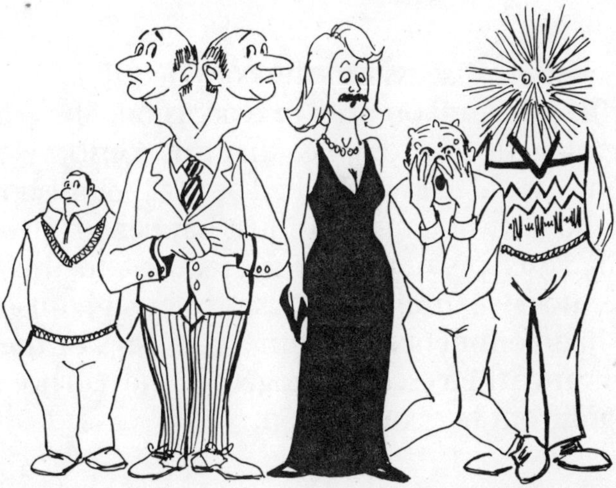

One Saturday evening while I was on call at the hospital, I was called to the Emergency department to see a thirteen year old girl who was being assessed for severe pain in her lower abdomen. I was extremely tired as I had had no sleep the preceding night due to the arrival of four new bundles of joy, and I had been working all day. Somewhat emotionally and physically drained, I proceeded down to the Emergency area to meet this frightened, shy, young lady.

Despite her stoic efforts to hide the obvious discomfort that she was feeling, it was obvious that our young patient was in pain and had a fever. She had already been assessed by a nurse, the Emergency room physician, and then had been examined by a general surgeon. She was very soft spoken, reluctant to talk and gave an unclear and incomplete story. After finding out about the pain she was having, I attempted to get some background information regarding her menstrual cycles and her sexual history to see if there may be anything in her story that might point us to the cause of her illness.

After some discussion, she confided that she had slept with a 'friend' on only one occasion. She related in an apologetic tone of voice that this consort was an eighteen year old fellow who had been a lifelong bosom buddy and that one night 'It' just happened. She had never had sex previously or subsequent to this one episode and it was unlikely that she was pregnant as her period had commenced within a few days of the encounter. Since their escapade together, she had not seen nor heard from her companion.

Upon physical examination, she proved to be exquisitely tender on examination and both the surgeon and I were concerned that she was developing a serious problem. After putting her story and the findings together, it was still difficult to determine the exact cause of the problem. The surgeon felt that she might have a ruptured appendix, and I was unable to rule out the possibility of a serious problem involving her pelvic structures. In order to determine the source of the problem, it was necessary that we perform a laparoscopy, an operative procedure whereby we look directly into her abdomen with a visualizing instrument. As I tried to explain the hows and whys of the procedure, the young girl cried with loneliness and fear. And then, because she was under the age of eighteen, I spent the next hour and a half trying to locate her mother to get consent to do the procedure.

At the time of laparoscopy, I found a severe pelvic infection which turned out to be the result of gonorrhea. Her reproductive organs were extensively damaged and as I looked down the scope I wondered if, and how, I would tell this thirteen year old girl that she might never be able to naturally conceive a child because of that one encounter. While this young lady was anesthetized with me staring at her distorted pelvic structures, I wondered where her 'friend', who had passed this infection on to her, might be. It seemed grossly unfair that she be victimized by such devastation. This patient, however, is not alone. She is just one of many women, throughout the world, who suffer as a result of STDs.

Listing all the possible complications of STDs would be both tedious and boring. It is important, however, to emphasize that as gynecologists, many of the day to day problems we encounter in our offices, are the result or complication of an STD. These include chronic pelvic and abdominal pain, pain with intercourse, infertility, vaginal discharge, abnormal pap smears, ectopic pregnancy, and abnormal genital growths, not to mention the psychological stress endured by many. It is also important for people with these kinds of complaints to realize that these concerns are often the result of other problems completely unrelated to STDs. Those afflicted with STDs, however, frequently do seek treatment for these complaints.

Some of the physical problems associated with certain STDs have received much attention. The well publicized complication of prolonged illness and eventual death often associated with HIV has been covered extensively by the media. The identification of cancer of the cervix, and many of the cancers of the vulva and vagina as a complication of HPV is gaining more and more support within the research world. There are, however, emotional and psychological burdens inflicted by STDs. Knowing that one has ongoing or recurrent carrier status, with the ability to transmit infection and illness to sexual partners, often has serious repercussions on healthy sexual relationships. Finally, the stigma felt by individuals with certain types of STDs may have significant emotional impact.

In addition to the physical, emotional, and psychological cost felt by many individual patients with STDs, there is also an enormous cost carried by society. It is difficult to accurately assess financial cost associated with these illnesses, but as an example, it is estimated that the cost of pelvic infections and the subsequent complications of tubal infertility and ectopic pregnancy exceeds $2 billion dollars per year in the United States[1] and many millions in Canada. This figure does not include the cost of dealing with HPV associated genital cancers, the medical therapies and palliative care required to victims of AIDS, and the psychotherapy, counselling and support provided by health professionals to those afflicted with STDs. All totalled, the sum, which continues to escalate each and every year, is staggering. In Canada, where most of the medical costs are incurred by the government funded health care system, this additional financial load is certainly stressing an already burdened health plan.

There is concern as to how the health care system is going to sustain the costs of providing for the needs of those afflicted with the HIV infection. As these productive, often young, taxpayers become disabled with sometimes long and protracted illnesses, funds will need to be generated to provide for their medical requirements. If the numbers infected continue to rise significantly, as many predict, insurance companies will also be challenged as disability and life insurance plans are redeemed. In some countries, the very social and political infrastructures are threatened as large numbers of people are affected by the disease. For example, this concern is apparent in Zimbabwe where the head of National AIDS Council stated that 58% of the people dying of AIDS come from the skilled professional class.[2] Furthermore, a report from this same country indicates that 90 per cent of the workforce could be HIV infected in 10 years time.[3] Some have said " ...the AIDS epidemic carries the potential to be the greatest natural tragedy in human history".[4]

The personal economic cost to individuals and couples is also exorbitant. A young couple recently came to my office because of their inability to have children. After thorough investigation, the woman was found to have extensive pelvic scarring as a result of a Chlamydial infection that she had acquired many years prior to her marriage. She had developed an ectopic pregnancy requiring an urgent operation and subsequently never conceived again. This couple desperately wished to have a child and opted for attempting in-vitro fertilization— a new reproductive technology. After mortgaging their home, they spent close to twenty thousand dollars on the required medication, travel expenses, and three attempts at the procedure itself. The repeated failures resulted in severe psychological trauma as the young woman rode an "emotional rollercoaster" with the repeated anticipation of becoming pregnant and the subsequent failures. She finally gave up on the attempts, on her marriage and almost on herself. Similar cases occur daily and it is not hard to imagine that in addition to the economic costs, the emotional complications of STDs can be horrific.

At a recent conference on the topic of infertility, much comment was made on the explosion in research surrounding assisted reproductive technologies. There have been, and continues to be, countless millions of dollars spent worldwide to find new ways to assist infertile couples. Through this concerted effort, there have been a few thousand children born via the in-vitro fertilization method over the last decade. Over the same period of time, however, there have been hundreds of thousands, or even millions of women who have acquired the problem of infertility as a result of sexually transmitted infections that they have contacted at some point in their life. One speaker expressed passionate frustration that the medical world continues to be misdirected with a focus on "...treatment, treatment, treatment..." rather than concentrating on these preventable diseases before they strike.

It is evident that there are both serious and long term consequences affecting many individuals who have acquired STDs. When considering the physical, emotional, and economic risks associated with certain types of sexual behavior, one can only conclude that it is time for all people to become informed so that appropriate choices can be made.

In the medical world today , there are ever-increasing medico-legal concerns. At times, patients have unrealistic expectations of what physicians are able to accomplish. There is an expectation that everything be perfect and should this perfection not be realized, a source of error is often sought. Accordingly, physicians have been encouraged to obtain "informed consent" from their patients. This is simply an effort to clearly educate patients regarding the potential benefits and complications, the success and failure rates, and all the ramifications of any proposed treatment or procedure. This educational process assists the patient, and his or her family, in making clear and appropriate decisions about treatment. Without this information, it is not possible for an individual to make an informed choice.

As it is recognized that there are serious complications associated with certain types of sexual behavior and lifestyles, "informed consent" through education should apply in this area as well. I have seen numerous individuals in my office and at the hospital with the various STDs. It is usually the case that the infected individuals had neither heard of their disease nor were aware of their risk of contacting it.

Chapter #8

What About the Condom?

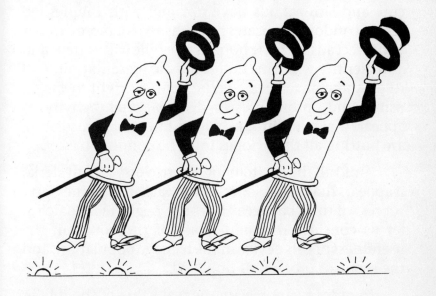

Over the last few years, the condom has been promoted as the method of choice for preventing STDs. It has been described as the "vaccine" against such afflictions, and condom use has been the mainstay of the so-called "Safe Sex" and "Safer Sex" campaigns. This inanimate object has received astounding notoriety and has been advertised on television and radio; it has been carried and promoted in elementary schools through to universities; and has been advocated by certain church groups, government institutions, and many experts in the medical profession.

There have been a variety of clever and witty advertisements with such catchy phrases as "Don't go out without your rubbers" and pictures of condom dresswear with the jingle "Evening wear for lovers that care." The condomania mentality is increasingly pervasive to the extent that I recently saw a novelty store advertising "Used Rubbers for Real Cheap Lovers!" As cute and shrewd ads have not met with the desired result, condom advocates have pushed for more explicit and direct ads with the hope that people will understand and identify with this more realistic presentation. As a result there have been a variety of forthright messages using crude profanities to discuss sexual activity. It appears that many groups, with influential sponsorship, are putting all their hopes into the condom basket.

Amid all the excitement, controversy and hysteria, it appears that a cold sobering look at the usefulness and success of this "panacea" has been neglected. To do so, let us consider the failure rate of the condom, the usefulness of this device in the teenage population, and the scope of protection provided.

In order to appreciate the real value of the rubber condom, it is first necessary to assess its performance in relation to preventing unwanted pregnancy. To define the success of any contraceptive method, the medical community has established a definition and standard by which each method is evaluated. The effectiveness of a given form of birth control can be discussed in terms of its 'Theoretical Effectiveness', and its 'Practical' or 'Actual Effectiveness'. The Theoretical Value is the potency under so-called ideal conditions with no defects, omissions, or improper use. The Practical Value is the success achieved at preventing pregnancy in real life with real people. As our current world is made up of real people, we will deal with the Practical Effectiveness.

The effectiveness of a contraceptive method is defined in terms of the phrase "number per 100 woman-years." This definition is designed to complete the sentence:

> **"Of 100 typical users who start out the year employing a given method of contraception, the number who will be pregnant by the end of that year will be _____."**

After reviewing the extensive literature on contraception, some variation in results is found. Reported failure rates for condom use vary from about 2 to 35 unplanned pregnancies per year, but a conservative consensus reveals a rate in the range of 8 failures per 100 users each year in the general population. Simple mathematics would conclude that after five years, the number pregnant with this method would be five times the yearly rate. Thus, after five years of condom use, there would be about forty pregnancies in this group of 100 real people; after ten years there would be eighty pregnancies. The two tables [8-1 & 8-2] are examples of charts depicting failure rates of various forms of family planning.

Table 8-1

First Year Failure Rates of Birth Control Users[1]

Method	Failure Rate in Typical Users
Tubal Ligation	0.04
Vasectomy	0.15
Combined Birth control pills	2
IUD	4
Condom	10

Table 8-2

Percent of Couples Who Experience Contraceptive Failure within the First Year of Contraceptive Use[2]

Method	Failure
Oral Contraceptive	2.0
IUD	4.2
Condom	10.1
Diaphragm	13.1

Despite much effort and money directly aimed at educating teens about birth control, there is a dramatically higher failure rate in this population. For example, the oral contraceptive medication has a Practical failure rate of about 1-2% per year in the general population, but a major study on contraceptive failure reported that in single woman under 18 years of age, using the birth control pill to prevent pregnancy, the first year failure rate was 11%![3] The failure rate of condoms is also seriously higher in the adolescent age group. For example, an article in the journal, Family Planning Perspectives, quotes an annual Practical failure rate of 18.4 percent in teenage girls under 18 years of age who are using condoms to prevent pregnancy. According to these figures, over half of the teenage users will be pregnant within three years. The authors further qualify this failure rate by stating that "these rates are understated because of the substantial underreporting of abortion among single women; if abortion reporting was complete, failure rates would be 1.4 times as high as they appear here..." [4]

In an attempt to defend the usefulness of the

condom, some have suggested that it might be easier to get pregnant than to catch a STD. How valid is this claim? In the normal reproductive cycle, which lasts about four weeks on average, the human egg is fertilizable for only 12-24 hours.[5] Sperm generally retain their ability to fertilize for 24-48 hours [6,7], although they may live for a longer period. There are thus, on average, only three to four days per cycle when sexual intercourse may result in conception. Conversely stated, normal physiology dictates that it is usually not possible to conceive a pregnancy for 85% of the year regardless of the sexual practices of those involved. Furthermore, in any given month, intercourse during this fertile time results in a viable pregnancy only about 20% of the time on average. This illustration would suggest that the high failure rate of condoms, with such a short available time for conception to occur, places this rubber saviour in a poor light in preventing unplanned pregnancy. The concerning point is that sexually transmitted diseases can be contacted at any time of the year and at any time of the menstrual cycle.

This limited effectiveness in preventing infection has been addressed in an article in the New England Journal of Medicine entitled "What is Safe Sex?" . The author comments in reference to AIDS, "It is clear that the use of condoms will not eliminate the risk of transmission and must be viewed as a secondary strategy."[8]

Some have tried to support the condom mentality to prevent the spread of AIDS by pointing to a transient reduction in the very significant incidence of gonorrhea in certain groups after encouraging condom usage. This is a rather tenuous premise as HIV and gonorrhea are totally different. "Unlike gonorrhea, HIV infection cannot be cured, is certain to be carried for a long time (possibly for life), and is highly likely to cause death. The risk of transmitting HIV must therefore be eliminated, since there is no acceptable level for this risk."[9] Furthermore, there is mounting evidence that since 1988, the incidence of gonorrhea has been rising.[10]

Another very significant shortcoming of the condom is illustrated by two of the common viral STDs. Both the human papilloma virus (HPV)(which has recently been closely linked with genital tract cancers), and the herpes simplex virus, are not confined to the localized areas under the often-thought omnipotent protection of the condom. They are frequently found in various locations of the external genital tract (e.g. vulva, clitoris, anal and groin areas). As intercourse generally involves contact in these regions, it is apparent that condom usage would provide little, if any, protection against these types of organisms. As has been mentioned, this is particularly disturbing when one considers that there is at least a 50% chance of transmission of HPV with a single sexual encounter with an infected person.[11] The abysmal failure of condoms in this regard can be witnessed by the recent explosion in human papilloma and herpes simplex viral infections despite increased condom use.

In order to justify the continuous funding and promotion of condom education, it has been suggested that the high failure rate with condoms is most frequently due to improper use rather than condom malfunction. The Theoretical failure rate, or the rate which minimizes human error, has been stated as 2% per year. Accordingly, the dramatically higher Practical, or Real failure rate, is felt to be due to some element of human imperfection. The prevailing "pro condom" lobby emphasizes that if we "educate, educate, educate!", people will feel more comfortable and adept at using condoms and thus the rate of failure, and consequently the rates of unwanted pregnancy and STDs, will diminish. To address this claim let us consider a few points.

An extensive review of the medical literature reveals a particularly noteworthy study which attempts to assess practical condom effectiveness in a select and "condom-educated" population. In order to be eligible for the study, the participants had to be highly motivated towards family planning, aged 25-39 years, married, and British subjects. After education by the British Family Planning Association, contact was maintained with the couples to determine results and propose conclusions. Even in this very select group of married couples, the failure rate was 4% per year, or 20 pregnancies per 100 women every five years.[12] With such a dubious success rate in this motivated, informed group, it appears naively optimistic to expect greater success with condoms in a vulnerable, adolescent population. This study supports my own experience in medical practice over the last number of years; I have seen hundreds of couples who have conceived a pregnancy despite meticulous condom use.

In addition, there is no consistent evidence that the condom propaganda blitz has resulted in a decrease in STDs. I noted with interest that an article written in the Reproductive Health Digest was titled: "STDS: They're ALL still going up".[13] When one listens to statistics presented about any apparent difference that the condoms are making, it is once again very important to remember that statistics can often be interpreted in a variety of ways and require careful and close scrutiny of the overall situation. For example, I was recently told that the rate of rise of one infection has declined in a specific localized population. On careful examination, however, it became apparent that a significant proportion of the population in that area had already been infected, leaving a smaller pool available for new infection. The numbers alone might, in this example, suggest that the rate of infection is diminishing, but the total picture reveals that the infection has already markedly infiltrated the population studied, leaving fewer persons available for an initial infection. The conclusions drawn would obviously differ depending on how this scenario was viewed and presented.

It is interesting to note that in areas with relatively high rates of known HIV infection, there has been a particular emphasis placed on the dissemination of information about condoms. Yet, even in these areas, evidence supporting the effectiveness of this educational strategy has not been produced. In fact, an abstract from the American Journal of Public Health highlights this concern.

Over a year when public health information regarding AIDS intensified, changes in perceptions and use of condoms in a sample of sexually active adolescents in San Francisco were examined. Although perception that condoms prevent sexually transmitted diseases and the value and importance placed on avoiding STDs remained high, these were neither reflected in increased intentions to use condoms nor in increased use.[14]

Fourthly, as has been discussed, condoms do not offer protection for diseases that are transmitted by skin to skin contact such as human papilloma virus and herpes simplex virus, frequently found throughout the genital area in infected individuals. No degree of condom education will curb the transmission of these organisms.

Finally on this point, I would like to consider an analogy as it pertains to this idea of securing results by improved and omnipresent condom education. In the general scholastic realm, despite the efforts of teachers to "educate, educate, educate!" the performance and examination results do not approximate 98-100% in most students. Even with excellent teachers, with researched and refined instruction methods, and with available extra tutorials and assistance, rarely do students achieve perfection. A few students score highly, most do average, and unfortunately a few fail. With condoms, however, anything less than perfection frequently results in the devastation of an unwanted pregnancy or a serious STD. One cannot help but question the expectation that with condom education most people will score near perfection. Yet, after a comprehensive review of the available literature on condoms, it is evident that the practical failure rate does not even come close to approximating perfection. To expect condom performance perfection, especially in teenagers where sexual activity is often unplanned, is grossly unrealistic—and this claim is supported by the disturbing escalation of STDs rates despite condom advertising.

An additional precaution that some have recommended to shield against STDs has been the "Coat of Armour" or the use of a spermicide in combination with a condom. While this supplement certainly decreases the rate of pregnancy, the toxic agents used to destroy the sperm may also have localized toxic effects on the body's own natural defense mechanisms. A concern was recently expressed that spermicide use may alter the protective lining of the vagina to perhaps more easily facilitate entry of HIV into the body.[15]

Over the last few years, there has been significant and increasing pressure to provide teenagers with easy access to condoms by placing dispensers in school washrooms. Let us consider two of the messages this undertaking provides to the students in schools harboring these machines:

1) **There is a serious problem with STDs and something has to be done to diminish this problem.**

2) **Condoms provide effective protection against STDs.**

Although the first message is absolutely true, the second suggestion is both dangerous and misleading. It provides people with a false sense of security-the mistaken notion that sex, utilizing a condom, is "safe". (The phrase "safe sex" has almost become synonymous with "using a condom during sexual activity".) If a condom is used, it is often assumed that sexual involvement carries no significant risk. As a result couples may engage in certain types of sexual activity that they otherwise might reconsider if the real hazards were known.

In general, it is important that inherent in any policy or program, there should be a mechanism to continually verify the real impact being made on people. This would ensure that programs based on hopes and projections would be monitored to assess actual results. In other words, programs should be evaluated by achievements and results, not promises and dreams. Thus far, I am not aware of any conclusive evidence revealing that increasing access to condoms actually decreases pregnancy or STD rates. Furthermore, there have now been anecdotal findings in some smaller communities that unwanted pregnancy rates have in fact increased since the placement of condom dispensers in the educational institutions. One explanation offered for this phenomenon has been the "kill two birds with one stone" mentality where users assume that the condom will prevent both STDs and pregnancy. As a result, the condom has replaced more effective forms of pregnancy prevention with a resultant increase in the number of unexpected pregnancies.

Although it is undeniably true that with any given sexual encounter, a participant is at less risk of contacting some types of infection with the proper use of a condom, it is equally true that over time, the sustained success at avoiding STDs by condom use is doomed to failure for many unsuspecting victims.

Many groups have been intrigued as to the evolution of AIDS prevention programs. Some critics, recognizing the limited effectiveness of the condom plan, have puzzled as to the persistent emphasis on this strategy. With reference to AIDS prevention programs, it has been explained that "The urgent nature of the epidemic is such that we have been recommending and implementing a variety of prevention programs based more on a reasoned hope than an established efficacy."[16] Although it is understandable that an epidemic such as AIDS, with all the serious ramifications, would result in formulation of prevention strategies based on "...a reasoned hope...", enough time has elapsed to recognize the failure of the condom propaganda blitz despite previous hopes along this line.

With the phenomenon of global media coverage, world attention is being directed at the horrendous numbers of AIDS fatalities and the explosion of HIV in Africa, Asia and South America. As in other locations world wide, condoms are generally presented as the best and the only realistic prevention against transmission of this lethal virus. Addressing this matter at the Seventh International Conference on AIDS in Florence in 1991, President Yoweri Museveni of Uganda stated, "In countries like ours, where a mother often has to walk twenty miles to get an aspirin for her sick child, or five miles to get any water at all, the practical questions of getting a constant supply of condoms or using them properly may never be resolved." According to this national leader, the answer for his disease stricken country lies in "a return to our time-tested cultural practices which emphasized fidelity and condemnation of premarital or extramarital sex."[17]

It has often been expressed that most, though not all, of the STDs are sexist in nature. HIV is an example which appears to have serious complications in both men and women. Yet, with many of the other types of sexually transmitted infections, it is frequently the woman who is victimized by the serious complications, including infertility, cancer of the cervix, and other chronic pelvic problems. A female family physician recently commented to me that if the male partner suffered the majority of the complications, "...the pseudo-protection strategy of condom promotion would not be in place" and that "more effective strategies and types of prevention would have been implemented years ago!"

One evening, a short while ago, my wife and I attended an outdoor theater festival. While listening to a string quartet perform Vivaldi, I stood close by a kiosk where volunteers were distributing free "information" about AIDS. The little booth was adorned with posters, in an assortment of languages and styles, pushing the message of safe sex through condom usage. A young male volunteer attempted to inspire the passersby on the need to be "comfortable and familiar" with condoms as the only protection against AIDS. One gentleman, walking by with his preteen son, was stopped by the volunteer and an information pack and a free condom were offered. The father responded that these types of diseases had nothing to do with him or his son because they were "straight". It concerned me that condoms were being presented as the solution to the AIDS crisis, but of equal concern was the fact that many individuals do not recognize that STDs are a threat, regardless of sexual preference.

To put the problem in perspective, the rate of increase of new AIDS cases in the United States, went from 9 percent in 1989 to 23 percent in 1990. Over this same time period, the rate of increase of new AIDS cases tripled in women! Without exception, every population group, including men, women, newborns, individuals involved in high risk activities, and those with no known risk factors showed an increase in the rate of new AIDS cases. [18, 19] The World Health Organization recently estimated that up to 5,000 people are newly infected with the lethal AIDS virus every single day![20] Furthermore, it has been suggested that in the very near future, the second leading cause of death in many North American cities for men in their twenties, and the leading cause of death for women between the ages of twenty and forty will be AIDS. As the length of time from infection to death is frequently in excess of seven years, it is apparent that many people succumbing to this disease contracted it during their teenage years. A presentation in the New England Journal of Medicine states that in couples where one partner was HIV positive "...condoms failed to prevent HIV transmission in 3 of 18 couples, suggesting that the rate of condom failure with HIV may be as high as 17 percent."[21] As it is now evident that many people have been infected with the lethal AIDS virus despite meticulous condom use, and that condoms do not provide protection against some other STDs, it is clearly of utmost importance that all people have access to truthful and complete information so that they can make appropriate health decisions. Access to full information and responsible personal choice within the law are, after all, important elements of a free society.

In conclusion, we are in the midst of a profound crisis and the situation is deteriorating. It is imperative that people be fully informed and educated about the facts and the issues. The strategy of encouraging condom use is not meeting its objectives. Yet, despite this lack of success, many continue to not only support the condom as the major warrior against STDs, but vociferously deny and oppose education which includes the serious shortcomings of condom use for so-called "safe sex". It is time to critically assess the effectiveness of this type of protection and to implement an alternate plan of prevention to curb the ongoing devastation in the lives of young and old alike.

Chapter #9

Can Any of These Diseases Affect Newborn Children?

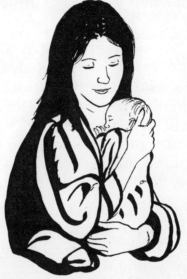

One Sunday afternoon, in my last year of training, a young woman was admitted to the labor and delivery area of the hospital having regular contractions. She had been seeing a doctor in another province from time to time during her pregnancy but was uncertain of her due date. On examination, she was found to be close to delivery and a general examination and history failed to reveal any impending problem. Within minutes of arrival in the birthing area, a vigorous, healthy eight pound baby was born. A week later, this newborn child was dead from a herpes infection.

The mother recalled in retrospect that three weeks ago she had developed an outbreak of sores in her genital area. She claimed the problem cleared up and for the last week she had not noticed any sores or discomfort. Because of the lack of symptoms, she assumed that she was perfectly well and at admission, when questioned regarding infections, she had not thought that her previous symptoms were of any consequence and thus denied any history of genital infections.

Herpes in the newborn child is a very serious disease. It commonly results in a central nervous system infection, with a resultant death rate of about 65% for untreated children. Of the survivors, less than 10% of these infants will develop normally.[1] Although Cesarean Section may prevent this tragedy if active infection is recognized, affected women may never realize that they have the disease if they have no symptoms.

Some of the STDs, such as syphilis, can significantly affect the child during development in the mother's womb. Other STDs, like herpes, can be contracted not only during the pregnancy but infection may also occur as the child passes through the birth canal. Another great concern over the last few years, is the fact that the newborn group has among the most rapid rate of increase for the AIDS infection. Tragically, in 1989, "...newborns got AIDS at a faster rate than gays or IV drug users."[2] The World Health Organization recently predicted that the AIDS virus will probably infect 10 million children by the year 2000![3] Unfortunately, there has been a need to establish pediatric AIDS wards in many hospitals in certain North American cities , just to attend to the ever increasing numbers of children with this affliction.

With some of the viral STDs, the impact of transmission to offspring has yet to be fully understood.

There has been some concern about the effect of the HPV infection on the developing child and research is currently being carried out in this area.

There are also many children who have acquired an STD as a result of sexual abuse. These innocent victims of both physical and emotional violence, may also have to suffer from the long term complications associated with these diseases. It is difficult to forget the evening I was called to Emergency to assess a three year old child who had been sexually molested by a member of her family. In addition to signs of trauma, evidence of gonorrhea was found in her genital area.

It is indeed tragic that many children have been made to bear the consequences for actions and decisions they have had no part in. At a time when many individuals are most vulnerable to STDs, in their teen and young adult years, most people have no idea that their actions may not only affect them, but may also result in profound complications for their future children. In the case of STDs, as in many other areas, the actions of parents will have an impact on their children.

Chapter 10

Are Teenagers at Any Special Risk?

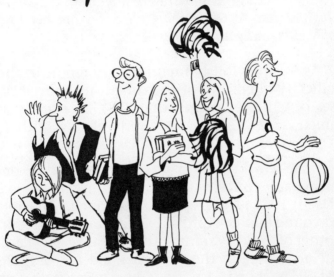

It is becoming increasingly more difficult and challenging to safely navigate through the teen and young adult years. There has been an escalating number of unwanted pregnancies with a resultant increase in abortion and single parent teen families. The suicide rate in adolescents is climbing at a frightening pace. There has been an alarming increase in drug and alcohol abuse that has resulted in the devastation of many families and a growth of associated criminal activity. Finally, we have begun to recognize the significant presence and serious effects of STDs and the profound impact they are having in our teenage population.

The problem of escalating STDs in adolescence is critical. The Brown University STD Update, June 1989 states:

The recent course of the AIDS epidemic has made a dramatic shift in the population affected, as has the changing course of other STDs. Statistics now show that populations at highest risk for developing all STDs are heterosexual adolescents and young adults, 14-22 years old.[1]

As was previously mentioned, a report in the December 1989 edition of the American Journal of Diseases of Children found that 38% of sexually active women, 13-21 years of age, were infected with a viral STD called Human papilloma virus.

The World Health Organization has expressed considerable concern regarding this growing menace of STDs. In 1989 , they reported that one in 20 teenagers and young adults worldwide will contract one form or another of sexually transmitted disease each year. They concluded that "... the growing incidence of AIDS and viral STDs, which are incurable, necessitate primary prevention of disease through promotion of behavioral change" and that "Public education is the only viable method now available to limit the extent of the HIV epidemic."[2]

It is imperative that this situation be addressed as sexually transmitted infections, once acquired, frequently have lifelong consequences. I recently saw a couple who, for over a year, had been trying to get pregnant. The woman's only previous sexual contact had been as a teen. Not long after her brief sexual relationship, this young woman developed genital warts, genital herpes sores, and was later diagnosed with a chlamydial infection. Prior to commencing sexual union with her husband, she consulted her physician as to how she might prevent transmission of these STDs to her loved one, and yet, at the same time, conceive a pregnancy. The patient claimed that she was instructed to have her husband meticulously use condoms, thus supposedly avoiding transmission of the HPV and herpes infections, and to cut a small hole at the tip of the condom to allow semen through in the hope of becoming pregnant. After twelve months, despite using condoms carefully with each encounter, her husband complained of having numerous genital warts and two recent outbreaks of herpes. Sadly, the young woman's tubal scarring from the previous chlamydial infection also has made it unlikely that she will conceive. It is evident that decisions made as a teen, have life-long ramifications for oneself as well as for future partners.

Although misconception and misinformation is not a problem particular to the adolescent age group, many of the woefully mistaken ideas about STDs are discovered in this population. Over the last few years, I have had the opportunity to give many presentations to school classes as well as to adult groups. I have also had the opportunity to review various questionnaires and studies done on the adolescent population to assess their knowledge, both practical and theoretical, on sexuality and STDs. The abysmal lack of knowledge regarding STDs and the many misconceptions and misinformation are appalling. Many feel they are not at risk because disease "passes only during the menstrual period", "only gays are at risk"; "only older people get that stuff"; and so on. The major tragedy is that some teens are making fundamentally important decisions in the area of sexuality based on such incorrect ideas.

Many physicians and pediatricians that I have talked to relate a common theme that they find to be prevalent in adolescent thinking. It can be described as the "invincible" mentality of youth. Although a teenager may possess some knowledge about pregnancy or STDs, when they encounter these problems personally, they often relate the sentiment that "I didn't think it could happen to me!" Because it frequently seems to be adults who are cautioning them about a variety of dangers, teens may view the advice as an overreaction and therefore not applicable to them. In hopes of circumventing this problem, some groups have trained teens to give workshops to their peers with the unproven assumption that in this setting, adolescents are more likely to listen and learn.

It has now been reported by a number of researchers that sexual activity in teenagers is frequently associated with a syndrome of problem behaviors that include drug and substance abuse, school difficulty, and delinquency.[3] A recent study of young teenagers found that in comparing those who were virgins and those who were not, the teenage boys and girls who had previously ever had sex were more likely to have used cigarettes and alcohol, smoked marijuana, and tried other illegal drugs. They were also more likely to have been suspended from school, to have run away from home, and to have been arrested or picked up by the police. Furthermore, the nonvirginal girls were six times more likely to have attempted suicide. The study found that teenage girls who had never had sex were much less likely to feel lonely, to feel upset and tense, to have trouble sleeping, or to have considered hurting themselves.[4] This is noteworthy as virginal girls are sometimes portrayed as unhappy, repressed, and lonely. The authors are NOT suggesting that early sexual experience is the cause for these negative behaviors or emotions, but rather, that adolescents involved with sex are not only at risk for the serious consequences of STDs and unwanted pregnancy, but are also at significant risk for these other health endangering behaviors and emotions.[5]

There is also a pervading media influence on all groups in our society including adolescents. I recently read a report detailing the fact that the average teen in North America spends 3.5 hours each day watching television.[6] The amount of sexually explicit and implicit material presented in the media is overwhelming with very little reference made to the health risks of such activity. A study recently reported that each year television exposes the average person, ten years or older, to more than 9,000 scenes of sexual intercourse, sexual comments, or sexual innuendo, with 80% of these involving extramarital or premarital encounters.[7] Associated with this material is the idea that premarital or extramarital sexual involvement rarely has serious consequences and is part and parcel of normal romantic involvement. When one considers the amount of time spent from early childhood to adulthood watching this message, it is easy to understand why many teenagers have no appreciation or practical knowledge about the real risks of diseases transmitted by sexual activity.

The area of sexual decision making presents a very difficult challenge for impressionable young adults. Whereas in the past there had been a general consensus as to what was considered acceptable sexual practice, there now appear to be conflicting ideas as to what type of behavior is most appropriate and normal. Many people in our society request that all be tolerant of any differing behaviors and that none is necessarily right or wrong. In the name of freedom and pluralism, we are asked to embrace and accept most types of sexual behavior as within the scope of normality. Accordingly, many teenagers are unclear as to what is appropriate or expected in the area of sexuality. Society provides little or no guidance to teens and many are being taught that there is no right or wrong but only various alternatives to suit individual sexual expression.

It is commonly felt and widely expressed that adolescents have uncontrollable urges, impulses, and needs along a sexual nature and that it is perfectly normal for these feelings to be expressed. In fact, those not partaking are often embarrassed to admit it and may feel ridiculed. It seems that sexual activity in this age group connotes ideas of fun, machoism, adventure, triumph, intimacy, and desirability. Unfortunately, the ideas of unwanted infection and/or pregnancy are nowhere to be found until they occur. The problems with drugs and alcohol appear to have exacerbated the situation. Under the influence of these agents, the capacity to make decisions may be altered and individual teens may succumb to behavior that they might otherwise not choose. As one pregnant teenager recently told me "If you're drunk, you just kind of forget."

Advertising programs aimed at reducing usage of alcohol by teenagers, with the display of the negative consequences of inappropriate alcohol use, is generally met with praise and admiration. Attempts to curb and prevent use of drugs in adolescents by emphasizing the clear realities and consequences of drug use are welcomed and encouraged by virtually all of society. Yet, effort aimed at diminishing teenage sexual activity, by clearly outlining the real and increasingly lethal consequences associated with such activity, is met with claims of moral interference. It is important that we do not let this serious problem be ignored and dismissed by some who would use the excuse of calling it a "moral issue."

How Do We Deal With the Problem?

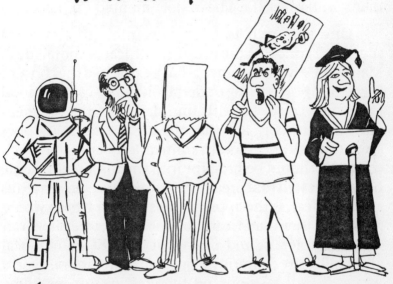

Although there appears to be general agreement that STDs are a very serious concern in our society, there is no clear consensus on a practical approach to solving the dilemma. It is therefore necessary that, after discussing the severity of the problem and becoming informed about the ramifications and potential complications, the possible solutions to the difficulties be addressed.

It is imperative that programs, developed to deal with a specific problem, be formally assessed to determine if they are successful or not. The success of a hockey team is measured by the score and whether or not the team wins, not by the number of good players, the team strategy, or the amount of money spent on salaries. In the same way, in order to assess the effectiveness of programs aimed at preventing STDs, it is necessary to observe if these approaches actually decrease the incidence of STDs, not how much money the government spends, the number of meetings held, or how many initiatives have been documented on paper.

One approach to STD prevention that is often suggested concerns the use of an ethical or moral ideal. Many conservative elements have expressed the concern that education is being undertaken in a so-called amoral (not to be confused with immoral) or values-free environment. Many feel that the area of sexuality does have ethical and moral ramifications and that such concerns should be brought into the discussion. Some have suggested that premarital abstinence, presented as a moral ideal, is the appropriate solution which would prevent rather than treat the problem. However, in our so-called tolerant and pluralistic society, many vocal and politically powerful groups interpret morality in a very different fashion and the conclusions regarding ideal sexual behavior are vastly different and often contradictory. The question then arises, whose morality do we choose? Many conclude that because of differing moral perspectives, an attempt should be made to educate with careful attention not to emphasize any moral inclination, thus leaving values out of the picture all together. But of course, teaching sexuality in the absence of values may be interpreted as a moral perspective all of its own.

Morals, and any laws for that matter, are important aspects of a free and healthy society. In an ideal world, legislation is developed and implemented to serve and protect individuals and communities. In other words, there are good and practical reasons to abide by, and uphold the law. In the same vein, to dogmatically present a moral perspective without a solid foundation as to the practical and documented benefits , is not likely to be fruitful in altering behavior, and leaves much room for criticism and ridicule. In the area of sexuality, it is truly sad that many organizations and individuals have been dismissed and ignored because their message of abstinence has been presented from a religious, moral, and dogmatic perspective without incorporation of the medical and physiologic benefits.

There are also advocates of a "Fire and Brimstone" approach to dealing with sexuality. Some groups and individuals have communicated the idea that people will suffer eternal damnation or be directly punished for transgressions of a sexual nature. However, on a practical level, this approach does not seem to diminish the transmission of STDs and some feel that it may well increase it. It appears historically that judgmental messages have not been an effective tool in altering sexual behavior.[1]

A couple of years ago, a well meaning individual was seriously concerned about the moral fibre of young people as well as the alarming rate of unwanted pregnancy. She had taken some courses and read books in the area of sexuality, and volunteered her services to educate young people. After her credentials were approved, she lectured to school groups at assemblies as well as to individual classes. A firm and moralistic approach was taken emphasizing the serious negative spiritual repercussions of engaging in premarital sexual frivolities. The results were disastrous with some very unfortunate consequences. The teachers reported that students were completely "turned off" and mocked and ridiculed the message. Furthermore the students were definitely adverse to hearing any further presentations on the topic and many subsequently scorned the idea of adults educating them about sexuality.

Many educational approaches in the area of sexuality have been proposed. I recently heard a politician suggest that, because of the very real and serious consequences of early sexual involvement, a campaign be presented to "scare the hell out of them". In this way he felt that teens would be frightened of sexual activity until they were old enough and mature enough to make appropriate decisions. This approach is countered by the philosophy of some who believe that the negative and harmful aspects of sexuality should not be discussed with young people in case "fears and phobias" are created which affect or impair normal sexual expression.

Another strategy is one which I like to term "the ostrich approach". Individuals may feel that their lack of sexual education was not detrimental to their lives and thus wonder why teens today require anything different. However, with the present inundation of sexual issues in the media , the entertainment market, and in general conversation, it is unlikely that many young people will have their heads "buried in the sand". They will receive information in this area from some source regardless of attempts to shield them, and thus it is important that the message presented be accurate and originating from a responsible source.

There are a large number of people who sincerely believe that attempts to modify sexual behavior are futile and naive. I have heard many health professionals and politicians indicate their belief that nothing can be said or done to stop individuals, particularly young teenagers, from participating in sexual activity. For this reason, they feel that encouraging universal condom use is the best solution that is realistically possible. Although they recognize that condom usage has serious limitations, these advocates often indicate that "there is nothing else that can be done!" Studies in this area, however, do not at all seem to support this fallacious idea.

If behavior modification can not be accomplished by appropriate suggestion and direction, why do parents and teachers spend countless hours educating, directing, counselling, and motivating children and young adults? If behavior modification can not be accomplished by appropriate suggestion and direction, why do advertisers continue to spend billions of dollars annually with the attempts to do so? I recall how, as a young boy, I would view beer and automobile advertising during the commercial time of televised hockey games. There can be only one reason why, twenty-five years later, the advertisements and promotions are still there. They are obviously successful in directing people to buy these products. As an executive of a liquor company recently mentioned in private, "It's not how it tastes or how good it is, it's how we market it!"

There are numerous people in our society, from individuals employed in marketing, to political lobbyists and strategists, whose job it is to influence opinion and effect behavioral change. Despite the reluctance of many to admit it, we are all influenced by what we see and hear. Why then, are people so convinced that accurate, reasonably presented information, will have no impact in the area of sexual behavior?

The most direct support for this ability to alter sexual behavior involves a study reported in the Journal of the American Medical Association in June, 1987 entitled 'Reducing Adolescent Pregnancy Through School and Community-Based Education'.[2] The study assesses the success of intervention programs in reducing the incidence of unintended pregnancies in the un-married adolescent population of a portion of a South Carolina County. A direct attempt was made to modify behavior in this group and the results were reported not by summaries of nebulous questionnaires or subjective attitudes, but in actual pregnancies.

The primary behavioral objective of this study was to postpone initial voluntary sexual intercourse among never married teens and pre-teens. The educational objective was to promote the postponement of initial intercourse as the positive, preferred health decision. The western portion of the county was involved in the program, and the results were compared to the eastern portion of the county and to three sociodemographically similar counties. The results are remarkable. After intervention, the pregnancy rate in the western portion of the county declined by about sixty per cent whereas pregnancy rates in the three non-neighbouring comparison counties increased. This approach is particularly remarkable when compared to many contraceptive based sex education programs that have provided little evidence of reduced sexual activity, of diminished teenage pregnancy rates, or of increased effective contraceptive use.[3]

This project in the South Carolina county, that quickly effected a dramatic reduction in the number of unplanned pregnancies, is worth looking at. I think this model of intervention provides the best route to quickly and efficiently decrease the upward spiral of STDs.

COMMUNITY RECOGNITION OF A SOCIAL PROGRAM

Training & Education of Adult Leaders

Teachers   Religious Leaders   Parents   Community Agencies & Professionals

Education programs for Youth and Families in Schools, Churches and Community Agencies [4]

In this model, responsibility is shared not only by the government and the medical community, but families and the community have a pivotal role as well. In the South Carolina county where it was implemented, this approach was remarkably successful at minimal cost.

If we hope to make progress in combatting the universal problem of STDs , it is important that all elements of society be adequately educated. There is widespread ignorance which is not just confined to young people. Accordingly, methods have to be identified to educate adults as well as the teens. Attempts have been made to educate teens through instruction at the school level without involvement of parents and the remainder of the community. This limited approach does not appear to have a sustained effect at modifying behavior. A significant decline in knowledge and a lack of behavioral change are noted after a short time has passed. It did appear, however, that personal lectures presented by health professionals directly to the students, resulted in a longer retention of the information than occurred when students passively received the information from a film.[5]

So what should be done in our cities and rural areas to make a positive impact on the epidemic of STDs? Regional medical associations, with support and commitment from the department of health, should assign a physician medical director to plan, direct, implement and monitor an educational program. Under the auspices of this medical director, a team of health professionals should coordinate and implement the training and education of adult leaders such as public health nurses, sexuality educators, school trustees, etc., in the various communities. This may be undertaken with community seminars or recurring workshops. As the community leaders become cognizant of the problem and the need for intervention and prevention, communication with the general community would then be required. These teams of adult leaders would coordinate efforts and be responsible to ensure adequate dissemination of materials and information to their designated community. Through their contacts and influence, educational seminars would be designed involving the team of health professionals and the medical director. These professionals would make presentations to the community at large through the school system, and through various community groups and agencies.

The main objective of the curriculum should be to present honest education incorporating all perspectives on the issues. Topics addressed should include STDs, unwanted pregnancies, pros and cons of condoms and other protective methods with failure rates and other limitations. The fundamental idea that sexuality is an important, wonderful, and healthy component of normal living should be communicated. Within this context, the message to postpone initial voluntary intercourse as the appropriate health decision should be forwarded to teens. Rather than portraying appropriate health decisions as repressive or restrictive, these lifestyle decisions and behavioral changes must be promoted as "life-sustaining and life-enhancing, as behavioral changes based solely on fear are not likely to be long-lasting." (Quoted with permission from a conversation with Dr. L. Jewell, previous Chair of AIDS Network of Edmonton)

Recognizing that the risk of contacting STDs, including AIDS, increases substantially with each additional sexual partner, the appropriate health decision forwarded should be long term monogamous relationships. As certain types of sexual activity, such as anal intercourse, appear to be correlated with a much higher risk of some types of STDs, these activities should be discouraged from a health perspective. (This specific example is not in keeping with the current trend in some circles which encourage anal intercourse to avoid the risk of pregnancy.)

Equipped with the information, individuals would then be free to make their own personal choices, a right that we so cherish in our democratic society. Some have claimed that the AIDS epidemic carries the potential to be the greatest natural tragedy in human history. But without the available knowledge and information about such a disease, it is impossible for a person to make an appropriate and informed personal decision.

It is naive, however, to suggest that all people will make healthy lifestyle decisions. Many people abuse alcohol and drugs despite abundant evidence clearly outlining the risks. For individuals who, despite education and understanding, choose to place themselves and others at risk for STDs, meticulous condom use will decrease the risk of contacting some, but not all, of these diseases. Adequate education programs should also enable those who are already infected to take appropriate measures to diminish secondary complications or spread where possible.

It is important that didactic traditional medical lectures or judgmental dissertations be avoided. I have found that when medical and social fact are combined with relevant case scenarios, both the interest and long term recall of the audience is enhanced. This also assists people in understanding how these infections relate to real people in their own environments and communities.

From an economic perspective, the cost of such a program to prevent STDs pales in comparison to the financial cost of assessing, treating and maintaining individuals who become victims of these diseases and their complications.

Interested and concerned citizens must accept responsibility and become a part of the solution. There is much that can be done in individual communities that will not only affect long term societal change, but will also make a difference in individual lives. Teachers and educators, once equipped and familiar with the information, can then promote frank and open discussion in the classroom. Some teachers and parents have chosen age appropriate chapters, sections, or stories from this book to stimulate lively and important discussion with their students and children. Professional development days for educators, in-services for social service and health personnel, symposiums for government officials, and communication within the memberships of various non-governmental organizations can all be used as occasions to introduce the concerns about STDs and to educate people. Finally, discussion of the STD problem and the need for education on an informal basis, with friends and neighbours, is a vital component of raising awareness.

It is my feeling that health professionals also have a responsibility to reinforce the STD concern to any patients or clients who are at risk. For example, when an individual comes in for contraception to avoid pregnancy with a new partner, it is my belief that a discussion regarding STDs should be part of the visit. If the patient is not aware of the reality of the problem, which is most commonly the situation, how can he or she make an intelligent and informed decision?

Some suggest that, rather than concentrating on the risks of STDs, it is more positive and appropriate to encourage "responsible" or "safe" sex using "fun" and explicit teaching methods. There are those who oppose the presentation of the reality of STDs by labelling it as "sensational" or as using "scare tactics". Many of these people conclude that condoms are the primary and only sensible and realistic answer to the problem of STDs. However, rather than attempting to be "sensational" there are three basic messages which underlie the approach as stated in this book: i) Sexuality is a wonderful, healthy, normal part of life. ii) Sexually transmitted diseases are a serious problem. iii) Individuals in our society are at personal risk for infection. It is the perspective of this book that presenting the whole truth , including the reality of STDs and the pros and cons of condom use, is closer to the answer. It is certainly my view that full knowledge is liberating and incomplete information is dangerous.

There will always be critics and vocal opponents to any strategy, no matter how effective and no matter how sensible. By the same token, there will be many who will not want to participate in workshops or training. But in my experience, there are a multitude of parents and community leaders that are keen to get involved and to positively effect change in our society.

In review, my suggested approach is that of education and recommendation. It is based on the medical model used daily by physicians in their offices. When a patient has a problem, we attempt to educate them about their illness, discussing causes, prognosis and treatment. The various alternatives for therapy including the risks, potential benefits and complications are discussed. After the alternatives are presented, patients are generally given a recommendation that their physician believes is the preferred and best health decision. Equipped with the education and direction, the patient is then informed and thus truly free to make a personal choice. The same phenomenon is true in the area of sexuality: comprehensive education empowers people to make wise decisions.

Chapter #12

Concluding Thoughts

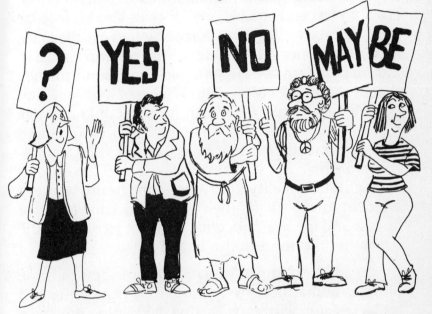

One of the most common questions asked is "If the problem is so bad, why are we not hearing more about it?" It is very difficult to adequately respond to this question but some of the answer is evident on close examination.

To begin with, the vast majority of people, including health professionals, have no idea as to the severity of the problem. As I am actively involved in teaching medical students and intern physicians, I often have the opportunity to give presentations at physicians' meetings, referred to in the medical lingo as 'giving rounds'. I am continually astonished at how little is generally known about the escalating problem of STDs.

I recently had the opportunity to question a very bright, mature, young physician, in training to be a family practitioner, about her knowledge of STDs. I enjoy presenting clinical situations to intern physicians, to test and challenge their skills and knowledge in practical, realistic situations. She had excelled academically in her medical class, and her knowledge of minutiae and trivia was admirable. She proudly told me that she had done very well in this area of study and that she felt very comfortable with her level of knowledge regarding STDs. Beyond regurgitating back facts and figures, however, her cognizance of the societal problem as a whole was virtually nonexistent. I have found it a frightening reality that these young health workers, often at the peak of their academic knowledge of disease and medical concerns, have not recognized the serious implications in the area of STDs.

In addition, the information about some of these illnesses and afflictions appears to be expanding and under revision with each passing day. Unless one has a particular interest in this field, it is hard to keep up with the ever changing, voluminous amount of literature that is being published in the medical journals. Accordingly, it is easy to fall behind on the current developments and to feel somewhat inadequate in relaying information to peers and trainees. Furthermore, because some aspects of STDs involve ethical decisions regarding treatment, disclosure of information, public health protection, and other sensitive issues, there is often significant controversy in how best to approach varying clinical situations. This also makes it difficult for a practising physician or public health official to know how to instruct others.

Most children and young people in North America receive their formal education within the school system. Parents and adults on the other hand, frequently rely on the media to obtain new and ongoing information. Ideally, as well as providing entertainment, the news industry should diligently seek information, assimilate facts, and present the news in an unbiased, accurate fashion. The public would thus be informed and educated. But just as individual professors and lecturers transmit information from their own understanding and perception of the data, it is only natural that individual reporters as well as editors and senior staff have personal perspectives through which information is interpreted and processed. The resultant presentation to the public may thus not portray a complete perspective.

In the case of STDs, a tragedy of incredible proportion, our media should be bombarding people with the information, alerting us to the spread and epidemiology of the problems, informing us about the successes and failures of available and experimental treatments, and so on. I see the need to present information on this threat the same way as we might see information presented on an ongoing conflict that was threatening somewhere in the world. However, after repeatedly hearing unpleasant news, people understandably get tired of it and become disinterested. The ongoing saga becomes depressing and "does not sell newspapers". The news media may then respond to this lack of enthusiasm and focus their energies on popular areas of current interest.

But in all fairness, the media can only relay information that they receive. If the professionals, who are directly involved on a day to day basis are not relaying their concerns to the information providers, how can we expect them to spread and disseminate the news? One physician, specializing in problems related to various infections, recently expressed the sentiment that it would be dangerous for physicians to explicitly tell the media how serious the problem with STDs is, because "they would put the public into panic!"

Throughout medical school, I employed various aids (no pun intended) to help me remember important facts and concepts. I would like to leave the reader with a little mnemonic, **"ACT NOW"** to help highlight some of the important aspects of STDs.

The **"A"** refers to the often Asymptomatic nature of many of these infections. In other words, at early stages of the infections, many people have no symptoms and thus carry and transmit STDs without knowledge of the presence of these organisms.

"C" points to the variety of Complications that may occur.

"T" reminds us that there is no Treatment to cure many of the current STDs, and to emphasize that once acquired, many complications of the diseases have no curative Treatment.

The **"N"** highlights the Need for educational programs.

"O" is a reminder of the far reaching potential to affect the Offspring of afflicted people.

Finally, the **"W"** emphasizes the Widespread nature of the STD problem and that in order to curb the crisis, Widespread action is required. It is imperative that people become willing to talk about the challenges and solutions to the STD problem with their children, teachers, school boards and politicians.

A-ASYMPTOMATIC
C-COMPLICATIONS
T-TREATMENT LACKING

N-NEED EDUCATIONAL PROGRAMS
O-OFFSPRING AFFECTED
W-WIDESPREAD

Before concluding, there is one additional issue which I would like to raise. Most diseases in the current age afflict primarily individuals, although certainly the loved ones are emotionally affected and often involved in supportive care. The disease of AIDS, however, targets not only individuals but also has the unique horror of taking aim at family units. A married man who is infected, may infect his wife, with an estimated 30-50% rate of infection to any children borne to the infected mother. The remaining children, who have not been infected, may eventually be left as orphans. The physical, economic, social, and psychological ramifications to family life are staggering.

There is much controversy as to what is to come in the near future with regards to STDs and particularly the AIDS epidemic. There are a few within the medical profession who have attempted to raise public awareness of STDs and especially the impending AIDS epidemic. But even within the medical community some of these individuals have been met with scepticism .

This scenario is very reminiscent of one involving a physician named Ignaz Philipp Semmelweis, who lived in the nineteenth century. Early in his medical career, this young physician made the startling discovery that a very high percentage of childbirth related deaths were a direct result of the unhygienic practises of the attending physicians. At that time, the mortality rate for women delivering in hospitals was exceeding high. When he presented his findings as well as conclusive proof of his theory, he was ridiculed, ostracized, slandered and persecuted by his colleagues and the medical establishment.

It was only after his premature death, as well as the unnecessary deaths of countless women, that his theories were accepted. To this day, medical practise is indebted to his discoveries, and his philosophies of cleanliness are practised universally. In the same way, the seriousness of the STD problem is equally evident and yet many are trying to downplay and ignore the situation. The time has come for both professional and lay people to equip themselves through education. Armed with knowledge, they must then mobilize and effect positive change in our schools, communities, and the political arena to curb the tragic onslaught of the STD threat.

NOTES

CHAPTER 2

(1) Division of Sexually Transmitted Diseases: Sexually Transmitted Disease Statistics,1987. Issue No.136. Atlanta, CDC, 1988

(2) Berg AO: The primary care physician and sexually transmitted disease control. In Holmes KK, et al(eds): Sexually Transmitted Diseases, ed 2. New York, McGraw-Hill,1990, pp1095-1098

(3) Edmonton Journal, Dec 11,1989, pC4

(4) Johnson RE, Nahmias AJ, Magder LS, et al: A seroepidemiologic survey of the prevalence of herpes simplex virus type 2 in the United States . New England Journal of Medicine 321:7-12,1989

(5) Cates W Jr., Toomey KE: Sexually transmitted diseases: Overview of the situation In Nixon SA,(ed):Primary Care, Clinics in Office Practice 17(1):13,1990

(6) Sullivan-Bolyai J, Hull HF, Wilson C, et al: Neonatal herpes simplex virus infection in King County, Washington. Journal of the American Medical Association 250:3059-3062, 1983

(7) Jeffrey J.F: Human papilloma virus and lower genital tract dysplasia: driver or passenger? Society of Obstetricians and Gynecologists of Canada Bulletin 10(4):5-15, 1988

(8) Rosenfeld WD et al: High prevalence of human papilloma virus infection and association with abnormal Papanicolaou smears in sexually active adolescents. American Journal of Diseases of Children 143:1443-1447,1989

(9) Becker TM, Stone KM, Cates W Jr: Epidemiology of genital herpes infections in the United States: The current situation. Journal of Reproductive Medicine 31:359-366, 1986

(10) Stone KM: Epidemiologic aspects of genital human papilloma virus infection. Clinic Obs Gyn 32:112-116, 1989

(11) Centers for Disease Control: Syphilis and congenital syphilis—United States 1985-88. Morbidity and Mortality Weekly Report 37:486:489, 1988

(12) Schultz S, et al: Congenital syphilis- New York City, 1986-1988. Morbidity and Mortality Weekly Report, 38(48):825-829, 1989

(13) Ricci JM, Fojaco RM, O'Sullivan MJ: Congenital syphilis: The University of Miami/Jackson Memorial Medical Center experience, 1986-1988. Obstetrics and Gynecology, 74(5): 687-693,1989

(14) Rolfs R, Goldberg M, Alexander ER, et al: Drug related behavior and syphilis in Philadelphia: "sex for drugs." (Abstract). American Journal of Epidemiology 128:898,1988

(15) Piot P, Plummer FA, Mhalu FS, et al: AIDS: an international perspective. Science 239: 573-579, 1988

(16) Causse GY: Worldwide microbial resistance to antimicrobial agents. Sexually Transmitted Diseases 7:333-339, 1984

(17) The Edmonton Journal, Feb 26,1989

(18) The Medical Post Jan 10, 1989, p.22

(19) Chin, James, Current and future dimensions of the HIV/AIDS pandemic in women and children. LANCET 336: 221-224, 1990

CHAPTER 3
(1) Snyder RR, Hammond TL, et al: Human papilloma virus associated with poor healing of episiotomy repairs. Obstetrics and Gynecology 76:664-667, 1990

(2) Beutner RR: Human papilloma virus infection. Journal of the American Academy of Dermatology 20:114-123, 1989

(3) Rapini RP: Venereal warts. In Nixon SA,(ed):Primary Care, Clinics in Office Practice 17(1):127,1990

(4) Moss AR, Bacchetti P: Natural history of human immunodeficiency virus infection. AIDS 3:55-61, 1989

CHAPTER 4
(1) Davajan, Val: "Infertility in the '90's", 28th Mousseau Memorial Lecture, Edmonton Alberta, Oct. 24, 1990, 0900.

(2) American Health Consultants, Courts give no guidance for managing infected workers, AIDS ALERT 5(6):101-120. 1990

(3) American Health Consultants, Courts give no guidance for managing infected workers, AIDS ALERT 5(6):101-120. 1990

(4) Centers for Disease Control. HIV/AIDS Surveillance Report. Year-end ed. January 1991

(5) Hewens FE, (Ed): Prevention— an idea whose time has come. Reproductive Health Digest 1(2):1, 1987

(6) Hewens FE, (Ed): Prevention— an idea whose time has come. Reproductive Health Digest 1(2):1, 1987

CHAPTER 5

(1) The European Collaborative Study - Children born to woman with HIV-1 infection: natural history and risk of transmission. Lancet 1991; 337: 253-260

(2) Imagawa DT, Lee MH, Wolinsky SM, Sano K, Morales F, Kwok S, Sninsky JJ, Nishanian PG, Giorgi J, Fahey JL, Dudley J, Visscher BR, Detels R: Human immunodeficiency virus type 1 infection in homosexual men who remain seronegative for prolonged periods. New England Journal of Medicine 320:1458-1462, 1989

(3) Imagawa DT, Lee MH, Wolinsky SM, Sano K, Morales F, Kwok S, Sninsky JJ, Nishanian PG, Giorgi J, Fahey JL, Dudley J, Visscher BR, Detels R: Human immunodeficiency virus type 1 infection in homosexual men who remain seronegative for prolonged periods. New England Journal of Medicine 320:1458-1462, 1989

(4) Moss AR, Bacchetti P: Natural history of human immunodeficiency virus infection. AIDS 3:55-61, 1989

(5) T. A. Peterman, J. W. Curran: Sexual transmission of human immunodeficiency virus, Journal of the American Medical Association 256: 2222,1986.

(6) Mertz GJ, Coombs RW, Ashley R, et al: Transmission of genital herpes in couples with one symptomatic and one asymptomatic partner: A prospective study. Journal of Infectious Disease 157:1169-1175,1988

(7) Mertz GJ, Schmidt O, Jourden JL, et al: Frequency of acquisition of first episode genital infection of herpes simplex virus from symptomatic and asymptomatic source contacts. Sexually Transmitted Diseases 12:33-39, 1985

(8) Rooney JF, Felser JM, Ostrove JM, et al: Acquisition of genital herpes from an asymptomatic sexual partner. New England Journal of Medicine 314:1561-1564, 1986

CHAPTER 6

(1) Masters W, Johnson V., Kolodny R: Crisis: Heterosexual Behavior in the Age of AIDS. New York: Grove Press, 1988, p.141.

CHAPTER 7

(1) Washington AE, Arno PS, Brooks MA: The economic cost of pelvic inflammatory disease. Journal of the American Medical Association, 255:1735-1738, 1986

(2) The Edmonton Journal, August 8, 1990, p.2

(3) The Edmonton Journal, August 8, 1990, p.2

(4) Masters W, Johnson V., Kolodny R: Crisis:Heterosexual Behavior in the Age of AIDS. New York: Grove Press, 1988, p.11

CHAPTER 8

(1) adapted from Hatcher R.A., et al: Contraceptive Technology 1982-1983 (ed. 11) New York: Irvington Publishers Inc., 1982, p.5

(2) from Vaughan, B., et al.: Contraceptive failure among married women in the United States, 1970-1973. Family Planning Perspectives 9:251,1977

(3) Grady WR, Hayward MD, Yagi J: Contraceptive failure in United States: estimates from the 1982 National Survey of Family Growth. Family Planning Perspectives, 18(5): 200-209, 1986

(4) Grady WR, Hayward MD, Yagi J: Contraceptive failure in United States: estimates from the 1982 National Survey of Family Growth. Family Planning Perspectives, 18(5): 200-209, 1986

(5) Speroff, L, Glass R, Kase N: Clinical Gynecologic Endocrinology and Infertility. 2nd ed. Baltimore, Williams and Wilkins,1982, p.327

(6) Speroff, L, Glass R, Kase N: Clinical Gynecologic Endocrinology and Infertility. 2nd ed. Baltimore, Williams and Wilkins,1982, p.327

(7) Austin CR, Human Embryos, the debate on assisted reproduction, Oxford University Press, p.6 1989.

(8) Goedert, J J:What is safe sex? New England Journal of Medicine 316(21):1339-1341, 1987

(9) Goedert, J J:What is safe sex? New England Journal of Medicine 316(21):1339-1341, 1987

(10) Hewens FE, (Ed): Gonorrhea total-like its antibiotic-resistant variety-goes up. Reproductive Health Quarterly Fall 1990, p.1.

(11) Beutner RR: Human papilloma virus infection. Journal of the American Academy of Dermatology 20:114-123, 1989

(12) Glass R, Vessey M, Wiggins P: Use effectiveness of the condom in a selected family planning clinic population in the United Kingdom. Contraception 10(6):591-598, 1974

(13) Hewens F E,(Ed), STDS: They're ALL still going up, Reproductive Health Digest,1(4):1 1988

(14) Kegeles, SM, Adler NE, Irwin CE: Sexually active adolescents and condoms: changes over one year in knowledge, attitudes and use. American Journal of Public Health 78(4):460-461, 1988

(15) Kreiss et al: Efficacy of nonoxynol-9 in preventing human immunodeficiency virus transmission, V International Conference on AIDS, Abstract, p.54, 1989

(16) Cates W Jr: Reviews and commentary, Acquired immunodeficiency syndrome, sexually transmitted diseases, and epidemiology. American Journal of Epidemiology 131(5):755, 1990

(17) McConnell H: Africa, Asia, S. America, facing HIV explosion. The Medical Post, 27 (27):24, 1991

(18) Steel E, Haverkos HW: Increasing incidence of reported cases of AIDS. New England Journal of Medicine. 325(1):65-66, 1991

(19) Centers for Disease Control. HIV/AIDS Surveillance Report. Year-end ed. January 1991

(20) Heterosexual sex listed a cause in 75% of world's AIDS cases, Globe and Mail, Nov. 12, 1991, pA8

(21) Goedert, J J:What is safe sex? New England Journal of Medicine 316(21):1339-1341, 1987

CHAPTER 9

(1) Corey L, Spear PG: Infection with herpes simplex viruses New England Journal of Medicine 314:686-691, 749-759, 1986

(2) Cowley G, Hager M, Marshall R: Special Report on AIDS. Newsweek June 25, 1990 p.21

(3) The Edmonton Journal, Sept 26, 1990

CHAPTER 10

(1) McDonald CJ (ed): Health Education for the young needed to stop the spread of AIDS/STDs. Brown University STD Update, 2(8):8, 1989

(2) McDonald CJ(ed): Health Education for the young needed to stop the spread of AIDS/STDs. Brown University STD Update, 2(8):8, 1989

(3) Donovan JE, Jessor R. Structure of problem behavior in adolescence and young adulthood. J Consult Clinical Psychology 1985; 53:890-904

(4) Orr DP Beiter M Ingersoll G, Premature Sexual Activity as an indicator of psychosocial risk. Pediatrics Vol 87 No. 2 1991 p. 141-147

(5) Orr DP Beiter M Ingersoll G, Premature Sexual Activity as an indicator of psychosocial risk. Pediatrics Vol 87 No. 2 1991 p. 141-147

(6) Bonham GH, Clark M, O'Malley K, Nicholson A, Ready H, Smith L: In Trouble...A Way Out. Calgary Health Services, Calgary. p.55, 1987

(7) McDowell J: How to Help Your Child Say "No" To Sexual Pressure . Texas, Word Books Publisher p.28 1987

CHAPTER 11

(1) Brandt AM: No Magic Bullet: A Social History of Venereal Disease in the United States Since 1880. New York, Oxford University Press, 1985

(2) Vincent ML, Clearie AF, Schluchter MD: Reducing adolescent pregnancy through school and community based education. Journal of the American Medical Association 257(24):3382-3386, 1987

(3) Stout JW, Rivara FP: Schools and sex education: does it work? Pediatrics 83:375-379, 1989

(4) Vincent ML, Clearie AF, Schluchter MD: Reducing adolescent pregnancy through school and community based education. Journal of the American Medical Association 257(24):3382-3386, 1987 (adapted)

(5) Huszti HC, Clopton JR, Mason PJ: Acquired immunodeficiency syndrome educational program: effects on adolescents' knowledge and attitudes. Pediatrics 84(6):986-994, 1989

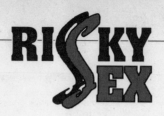

Additional copies may be ordered by sending $11.95 per copy plus $2.00 for the first copy and $.50 for each additional copy for shipping and handling. A discount is available on orders of 100 copies or more. Please make cheques payable to KEG Publishing.

Copies, orders or inquires regarding the book may be addressed to:

KEG Publishing
Box 32025
#420, 2331-66 Street
Edmonton Alberta
Canada
T6K 4C2

Telephone orders may be arranged by calling:
(403) 461-1606

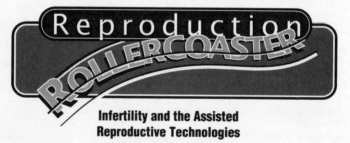

Infertility and the Assisted Reproductive Technologies

by Stephen Genuis M.D.

We have now reached the era where many view absolute control over reproduction as desirable, attainable, and the necessary key to truly achieve equality between the sexes. As was never before in the past, we can have sex without having children and have children without having sex. There are many who hail these developments as a blessing while others view this trend as a curse. It is my hope that the information presented will allow the reader to understand the problem of infertility, and to recognize and discern the ramifications of the assisted reproductive technologies that are flourishing all around us.

This important book will be available in the summer of 1992 from KEG Publishing.